Business Intelligence & Analytics: - A Hospital and Health Management Informatics Apparatus

Electronic Health Records [EHR] and the Future of Healthcare: A needed Technology Accelerator

Kwasi Yeboah-Afihene

[THIRD "SPECIAL" EDITION]

*Electronic Health Records (EHR) and the Future of Healthcare:
A needed Technology Accelerator.*

Copyright © 2015 by **Kwasi Yeboah-Afihene**

Library of Congress Control Number: Pending
ISBN-13: 978-1512251005
ISBN-10: 1512251003

All rights reserved. No part of this book may be reproduced or transmitted in any form or by any means, electronic or mechanical, including photocopying, recording, or by any information storage and retrieval system, without permission in writing from the copyright owner.

This book was printed in the United States of America.

Author's contact details:

kwasi_afihene@yahoo.com
kwasi.afihene@gmail.com
[Also on LinkedIn & Facebook]

Dedication

This book is dedicated to my Mentors, Faculty Advisers and Friends: Dr. Syed Haque (Rutgers University Biomedical Sciences – SHRP), Dr. Dinesh Mital (Rutgers University Biomedical Sciences – SHRP) and Dr. Shankar Srinivasan (Rutgers University Biomedical Sciences – SHRP), "The Entire SHRP – Health Informatics Department Faculty, Students and Staff". And also, Dr. O. Maillet: Dean of Rutgers University – School of Biomedical Sciences – SHRP & Staff, as well as all faithful readers.

BUSINESS INTELLIGENCE AND ANALYTICS: A HOSPITAL AND HEALTHCARE MANAGEMENT INFORMATICS APARUTUS.

(Health Informatics)

By

Kwasi Yeboah-Afihene

"Electronic Health Records [EHR] and the Future of Healthcare: A needed Technology Accelerator"

ACKNOWLEDGEMENT

I am thankful to the Almighty for his protection, and guidance for my life. I would also like to express my profound gratitude to my mentors at Rutgers University School of Biomedical Sciences – SHRP (Health Informatics Department), Dr Syed Haque, Dr. Dinesh Mital and Dr. Shankar Srinivasan. And also Dr. O. Maillet, the dean of SHRP.

To the brain-children of all related knowledge, I humbly say thanks for sharing. I will finally apologize to all direct and indirect contributors I missed in my personal acknowledgements. Please forgive me, and accept my apologies, and most sincere gratitude for all your good work, which I believe will serve and help many lead a healthy and quality life.

PREFACE

This book highlights the potentials of the Electronic Health Records [EHR] systems and their relevance as the most essential technology accelerator to thrust healthcare into the next millennium. It also contains a brief, integrated knowledge, which provides a broad overview of Business Intelligence and Analytics, as well as Healthcare Decision Support Systems, as they relate to Hospital/Healthcare Management. It highlights their importance and the industry's urgent need to incorporate requisite BI and Analytics technologies in their broad IT Strategy to help address, and resolve its most pressing issues; Some of which are related to operations, financial, administrative, customer satisfaction and regulations, and so on, to ensure healthy and positive outcomes across board.

Most of the ideas were drawn from a myriad of sources, including articles from professional periodicals and magazines. They are however presented in a multi-dimensional and integrative fashion, yet seamless to the reader, in its coherency. In other words, the story is told in a very professional way, with a heightened focus on its relevance to the industry and related stakeholders.

It will be useful to both clinician, and allied health professionals, as well as administrators and students. Healthcare leaders and managers will find it very useful as an overview of EHR, BI and Advanced Analytics. It is therefore a good starting point, for managers and leaders giving BI and Analytics a serious consideration in their overall strategic initiatives, whiles making considerations for EHR systems, [infrastructure and architecture] from which most of healthcare data emanate. The analysis of such data produce the needed actionable insights, which leads the way to the needed solutions to some or most of the problems facing the healthcare industry today and tomorrow. This edition is more concise and up to the point.

Table of Contents

PART I 20

Introduction 20

Healthcare/Hospital Information – Various Types 24

    Different views of Biomedical - Healthcare Informatics: 27

        View 1: 28

        View 2: 29

        View 3: 30

    Advanced Analytics: A discovery Mission 32

    Healthcare Portability and Accountability act's Definition of Healthcare Information 35

    National Alliance for Health Information Technology Definitions 36

- Healthcare Data Quality 38
- Healthcare/Hospital Information Systems 40
- Decision support Systems 42
  - Decision Support System – DSS 44
- Medical Decision Support Systems 47
  - Artificial Intelligence and Expert Systems 51
  - Medical decision support systems and the general nature of medical interventions 55
  - The two major distinctions of medical decision support systems 56
    - Intervention Types 58
    - Management Information Systems 59
    - Executive Information Systems 61
    - The Role of MIS 63

Accountable Care Organizations.....65

Business Intelligence and Analytics 68

BI and Analytics Vs Decision Support Systems.69

A brief Historical view of BI and Analytics 71

Technology Integration 74

Why BI & Analytics in Health Care? 76

    Healthcare Domains with Common Analytical Questions 78

    BI Competency Center 79

    The Basic Health Informatics Theory 80

    BI and the Electronic Health Records 82

    BI an integrated Summary View of Health Care Information 85

    BI – An Efficiency and Effectiveness Steroid..86

Basic Architecture 87

Targeted Outcomes for BI and Analytics Engagements 88

BI – Successes in Health Care 88

Interesting Issues 89

Advanced Analytics Adaptation Issues 90

Obstacles to BI Widespread Adoption 91

Problems or Opportunities 91

Other BI Momentum Drivers in the Healthcare Industry 92

Advanced Business Intelligence at Cardinal Health 94

Implementation Options and VENDORS 95

Section Conclusion 96

Big Data Applications in Health Care 97

MIT Sloan Management Review & IBM Institute For Business Value: Study Finding 102

Healthcare and Big Data 106

An Example of BI Implementation in Education: Penn State 108

Part II..125

MANAGING HEALTHCARE WITH DATA & RELATED BENEFITS...125

    Introduction 125

    Business Intelligence and Analytics 129

    A Brief Historical Perspective.........130

    BI AND BIG DATA: AN INTEGRATED VIEW..134

    BI – BIG DATA ANALYTICS: ADVANCED ANALYTICS 136

    Big Data Analytics...........................138

Interesting Adaptation Issues 138

Obstacles to Big Data Analytics Widespread Adoption 140

Problems or Opportunities 140

Big Data Applications In Healthcare 142

Health Care and Big Data 146

Potential Impact of Big Data on the Health Care System 150

Other Big Data Momentum Drivers in the Healthcare Industry 151

Outcomes: 151

Some Industry Wide Imperatives 152

Section Conclusion 153

PART III 155

IMPLEMENTATION EXAMPLES & CHALLENGES - [UK] 155

Initiatives..170

EHR & BIG DATA: - BASIC ARCHITECTURE [HEALTHCARE SUPPLY CHAIN AND REVENUE CYCLE]................................186

IDM & CDM Integration 189

Abrazo Health Care [CASE STUDY] - Study Findings..192

PART IV..199

PART IV..205

PART V...229

Electronic Health Records Incentive Payments for Eligible Professionals 234

PART VI..240

References 249

PART I

Introduction

Business intelligence and analytics, has emerged as the most formidable apparatus and ingenious decision making platform and aid in a myriad of industries. It has made a lot of strides and a great mark in many industries including the financial, insurance, marketing and sales, retail and so on. It has recently found its way in the healthcare industry.

From its onset till now, it has unleashed a lot of current and future potentials which has great benefit to the industry and its respective stakeholders. With the advent of the Big Data revolution, it has become even more valuable and a very essential component of any serious healthcare player's IT infrastructure and strategy. However not all the respective players have it in their arsenal. Not having it in the current or at least the immediate future IT strategy of any big player, is a recipe for extinction. For without it, a great competitive edge will submerge, leaving the organizations rabblements in the dust eventually. It other words it just cannot survive in the long haul.

Most healthcare players have however a heavy investment in legacy Medical Decision Support Systems which will inflict an immense financial pain, if it get to a point of discarding them totally, to rebuild a new robust system. It is great however to note that this need not be. The BI and analytic infrastructure can be built to integrate well with such Medical Decision

Support System, creating a more cost effective yet formidable tool to improve the clinical, operational and financial health of the organizations.

The apparent stresses that has plagued healthcare institutions on the clinical and care delivery side of the business, has created an emergency situation which has warranted an urgent need to act in favor of BI and Analytics. From financial to operational and capacity stresses on the systems today, I believe the stress test on them is almost at its climax, and inaction toward an immediate workable solution could spell doom. It is therefore a strategic imperative for these organizations to act with speed or plan their exit, which will just be in a matter of time.

This book is a review, which describes and highlights many of the pertinent issues and components of the BI & Analytics and MDSS, enlisting and explaining some of the requisite industry issues which the integrative system can help to alleviate, and consequently improve the performance of the players in the industry.

Healthcare/Hospital Information – Various Types

There is a myriad of healthcare information repositories classified by types. The various types of information are very pertinent to the clinical effectiveness as well as sound administration of healthcare systems. Some are generated internally; whiles others are of external origins, given the various stakeholders and vendors whose in-house data and information are sometimes very essential to the operational and administrative needs of such organizations. There are patient specific data and information, which is often very sensitive due to privacy laws such as HIPPA and other patient rights issues. However, desensitized aggregate patients, and administrative data are also very pertinent to healthcare institutions, for predictive, and outcome research purposes. The following are the various types of healthcare data and information:

- Internal Data and Information which is Patient Specific – Clinical
- Internal Data and information which is Patient Specific – Administrative
- Internal Data and Information which is Patient Specific – Combining Clinical and Administrative
- Internal Data and Information which is Aggregate – Clinical
- Internal Data and Information which is Aggregate – Administrative
- Internal Data and Information which is Aggregate – Combination of Clinical and Administrative.

- External Data and Information which is Comparative
- External Data and Information which is used for Expert or Knowledge Based purposes.

Different views of Biomedical - Healthcare Informatics:

From the article, "What informatics is and isn't" by Charles P. Friedman of Columbia University, he gave very interesting views of what Biomedical/Healthcare Informatics is and isn't. His views truly captured the multifaceted views of Informatics and disentangled the inaccuracies in some contemporary definitions by professionals in healthcare and others, mostly outside of the Informatics domain. The following is a summary of his views of what informatics is and isn't:

View I:

Informatics as Cross – Training: He viewed informatics as a cross training between the basic information sciences and some related application domains. Fig 37 illustrated the connection. "Informaticians" are neither experts in information science nor domain professionals like clinicians. They however have enough knowledge in both spheres to harness their potentials to enrich the industry's targeted outcomes. Such healthcare outcomes as; patient quality of life and satisfaction, financial sanity and so on are often improved significantly with the application of informatics processes and tools. They are therefore a bridge between the two.

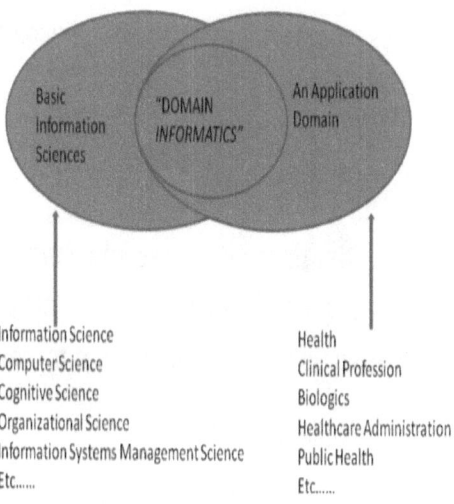

Information Science
Computer Science
Cognitive Science
Organizational Science
Information Systems Management Science
Etc......

Health
Clinical Profession
Biologics
Healthcare Administration
Public Health
Etc......

Figure 1

View 2:

The second view sees informatics as "a relentless pursuit of assisting people, as they work to improve health through appropriate use of information technology and conducting studies to determine whether the assistance has been successful".

View 3:

The third view sees informatics as steps in a sequence aligned with creating and evaluating an information system or resource:

1. Model formation
2. System Development
3. System Deployment
4. Study of effects

A comprehensive training in informatics therefore according to Friedman, is associated with understanding the ability to apply the science underlining the above steps.

Informatics therefore is neither of these exclusively, according to the article:

1. Scientist or Clinicians tinkering with computers
2. Analysis of large data
3. Circumscribed roles related to deployment and configuration of electronic health records in pursuit of meaningful use.
4. The profession of Health Information Management

Advanced Analytics: A discovery Mission

Advance Analytics is a collection of related techniques, process and tools, which usually include; predictive analytics, data mining, statistical analysis, and complex SQL. It also include, data visualization, artificial intelligence, natural language processing and database capabilities that support analytics. (eg. MapReduce, in-database analytics, in-memory databases, columnar data stores etc.

The main objective of advanced analytics is to sift through massive amount of variety of data to identify patterns and business facts which are yet to be discovered by either the industry or the company. These facts and insights support their strategic moves or solve major crippling problems, or sometimes improve operational efficiencies, or customer satisfaction. Ultimately these tend to improve sales and increase revenue and profits.

Big data discoveries mixed with historical data from the data warehouse, leads to a metric, report, analytic tools, or some other BI products to support decision making in the company. Advanced analytics can be enabled by different type of analytic tools, including SQL based queries, data mining, statistical analysis, fact clustering, data visualization, natural language processing, text analytics, artificial intelligence and a wide arsenal of tool which requires a savvy professional to access the needs of a particular organization.

Big Data:

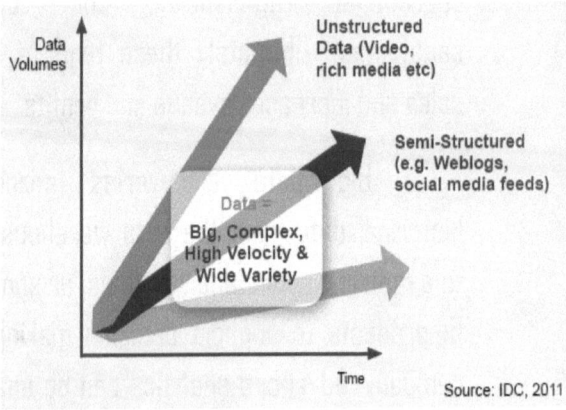

Figure 2

Big Data Analytics:

Big Data Analytics is where advanced analytics tools and techniques are used to operate on Big Data, to achieve the ends as have already been addressed previously in this document.

Healthcare Portability and Accountability act's Definition of Healthcare Information

Any information, whether oral or recorded in any form of medium, that:

- Is created or received by a healthcare provider, health plan, public health authority, employer, life insurer, school or university, or health care clearing house

- Relates to the past, present, or future physical or mental health or condition of an individual, the provision of health care to an individual, or the past present or future payment for the provision of health care to an individual.

National Alliance for Health Information Technology Definitions

- Electronic Medical Records: An electronic record of health related information on an individual that can be created, gathered, managed, and consulted by authorized clinicians and staff within one health care organization
- An electronic record of health-related information on an individual that

conforms to nationally recognized interoperability standards and that can be created, managed and consulted by authorized clinicians and staff across more than one health care organization.
- Personal health records – An electronic record of health-related information on an individual that conforms to nationally recognized interoperability standards and that can be drawn from multiple sources while being managed, shared, and controlled by the individual [Alliance 2008].

Healthcare Data Quality

Data is usually processed into information which is later translated to a useful knowledge which in turn can support various aspects of decision making within health care organization. "As the saying goes in information and computer sciences, garbage in garbage out". In other words, the quality of the data being collected is very crucial to the very end purpose. Poor quality data will therefore generate misleading knowledge which can create a disaster due to poor quality decisions. Quality data has the following characteristics as presented in the "AHIMA Data Quality Management Model:

- Accessibility

- Consistency
- Currency
- Granularity
- Precision
- Accuracy
- Comprehensiveness
- Definition
- Relevancy
- Timeliness"

AHIMA, Data Quality Management Task Force, 1998

Healthcare/Hospital Information Systems

Information Systems (IS) is an arrangement of information (Data), processes, people, and information technology that interact to collect, process, store, and provide as output, the information needed to support the organization (Whitten & Bentley, 2005) Information technology however is a description of a combination of Hardware and software, which constitute the infrastructure on which these systems run. (ie. Telecommunication Technologies, data, image, and voice networks, servers and the tons of applications that run on them). Health care Information Systems are simply information systems and related technologies that support a healthcare organization.

Decision support Systems

- Definition of decision support system in English (Oxford Dictionary)

  decision support system
  Syllabification: (de·ci·sion sup·port sys·tem)
  (abbreviation: DSS)
  noun
  Computing
  a set of related computer programs and the data required to assist with analysis and decision-making within an organization.

- A Decision Support System (DSS), is a computerized information system which is used by managers and employees of an organization to support their business decision making. It enables them to analyze and synthesise a lot of data and compile useful information that can be used to solve problems and make better decisions.

Decision Support System – DSS

"The benefits of decision support systems include more informed decision-making, timely problem solving, improved efficiency and better learning. A DSS can compile and present information for many aspects of a business, including sales trends, actual versus projected sales, worker productivity, and profitability mix and so on." (INVESTOPEDIA)

From Randall E. Louw's (University of Missouri, St Louis) article on Decision support Systems supervised by Prof. Prof. Vicky Sauter:, "…..Sprague and Watson (1996) conceptual models or frameworks are crucial to understanding a new and/or complex system. They define DSS broadly as an interactive computer based system that helps decision-makers use data and models to solve ill-structured, unstructured or semi-structured problems.

DSS provides varying analysis without much programming effort and is usually directed towards non-technical users/managers. Managers main uses for a DSS includes searching, retrieving and analyzing decision relevant data to allow them to summarize main points which assist them in making more informed and educated decisions. Users often search for correlations between data without rewriting the underlying MIS or software application and most DSS allows graphic capabilities, which not only allows trend analysis and reporting for top executives, but also assists managers in mapping out conjoint analysis and alternative scenarios to answer "what if" queries. Consequently, DSS supports both tactical and strategic decisions and are employed to leverage manager's expertise in a certain field." Ronald E. Louw, Prof. VickynSauter: University of Missouri, St Louis)

Medical Decision Support Systems

There are tons of data and information repositories in hospitals and other healthcare institutions in the country. These repositories are comprised of data accumulated over a period of time from clinical, operational and administrative routines, whiles others are real time data from patient monitoring devices. The human body alone comprises of a ton of data of which the clinically relevant ones are often generated during the clinical care delivery processes.

Most of clinical diagnostic processes generate a lot of relevant data about patients, examples of which are, patient lab work, medical images, recorded speeches, blood work and so on all have vital data and information about the respective patient. Patient vital statistics monitoring tools also generate a lot of data on patients depending on the organ or the sub system being monitored, be it the heart or brain etc.

Also administrative and operational data generated from the various business and job processes all produces a lot of useful data, some of which are used to streamline current operation, predict future trends and identify current and future opportunities of strategic essence.

Clinicians and other health care workers make several decisions about patients in the process of care delivery. Most of these are based on evidence as depicted in relevant data. Evidence based medicine recommends a health delivery process which is based on a critical analysis of empirical evidence, rather than reflective knowledge and experience alone.

The highly unstructured nature of medical operations and administration also warrants the need for such decision support systems, to improve the effectiveness and efficiency of their decision minimizing negative administrative outcomes that can have devastating consequences for the organization. With the mounting financial pressures and other resource scarcity in the health care system, the need to minimize errors due to wrong decisions has become even more critical. The technological basis for most medical decision support systems is Artificial Intelligence

Systems. They may either be Expert System or An Artificial Neural Networks Based. The next two sub topics will give brief explanation of the above technologies.

Artificial Intelligence and Expert Systems

A computer program that uses artificial intelligence to solve problems within a specialized domain that ordinarily requires human expertise. The first expert system was developed in 1965 by Edward Feigenbaum and Joshua Lederberg of Stanford University in California, U.S. Dendral, as their expert system was later known, was designed to analyze chemical compounds. Expert systems now have commercial applications in fields as diverse as medical diagnosis, petroleum engineering, and financial investing. In order to accomplish feats of apparent intelligence, an expert system relies on two components: a knowledge base, and an inference engine... (Encyclopedia Britannica)

Neural Networks:

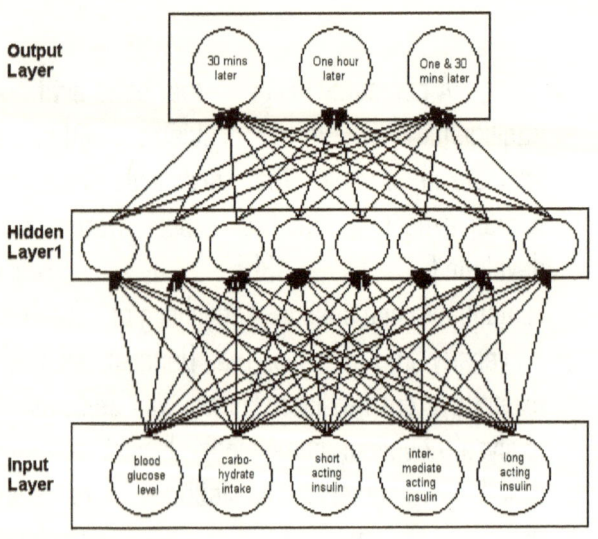

From: AIDA – Research Use(http://www.2aida.net/aida/research2.htm)

Figure 3

In computer science and related fields, artificial neural networks are models inspired by animal central nervous systems (in particular the brain) that are capable of machine learning in pattern of recognition. They are usually presented as systems of interconnected "neurons" that can compute values from inputs by feeding information through the network.

For example, in a neural network for handwriting recognition, a set of input neurons may be activated by the pixels of an input image representing a letter or digit. The activations of these neurons are then passed on, weighted and transformed by some function determined by the network's designer, to other neurons, etc., until finally an output neuron is activated that determines which character was read. Like other machine learning methods, neural networks have been used to solve a wide variety of tasks that are hard to solve using ordinary rule-based programming, including computer vision and speech recognition. Wikipedia: (http://en.wikipedia.org/wiki/Artificial_neural_network)

Medical decision support systems and the general nature of medical interventions

- Predict MDSS (Predictive Medicine)
- Prevent MDSS (Preventive Medicine)
- Heal MDSS (Curative medicine)
- Comfort Care MDSS (Medical Assistance)
- Patient Situation MDSS (Diagnosis and Prognosis)

The two major distinctions of medical decision support systems

A. In other to minimize the uncertainty in accessing patient's state, such systems access the prognosis and diagnosis of patient's conditions. These types of medical decision support systems consider information from varying disciplines such as:

    a. Epidemiology

    b. Semiology

    c. Pathology

    d. Physiology

    e. Anatomy and so on...

B. For formulating the right strategic care management and treatment, the second set of systems come into play, helping clinicians to determine what must be done. Such as:

    a. Which additional tests should be performed?

    b. Which medical images should be done?

    c. What medication or treatment should be recommended?

    d. The best way to counsel and inform patients and family about conditions.

    e. Financial and ethical considerations to think about in the care management process etc....

Intervention Types

Medical Decision support systems typically have three modes of operation:

- Passive Systems as in consultant and critical systems
- Semi-active Systems as in automatic reminder systems and Alarm systems
- Active Systems: they are triggered automatically to provide advice adapted to a particular patient. It can also automatically make decisions without the intervention of a physician (e.g. automatic control of a transfusion by a closed – loop system, Intelligent control of the parameters of a ventilator or a dialysis monitor or a pacemaker)

Management Information Systems

Management Information System (MIS) is a concept which has been out there for roughly two decades. It is quite young yet has been revolutionary in its application and usage. MIS is more of a concept which spans several definitions. Some of them are as listed below

- MIS is defined as a system which provides information support for decision making in organizations
- MIS is defined as an integrated system of man and machine for providing the information to support operations, management and other decision making function in organizations
- MIS is defined as a system based on the database of the organization evolved for the purpose of providing information

to the people in that organization.
- MIS is defined as a Computer based Information System.

In spite of the multi-dimensional views of the above definitions, they all converge however in summary, as a system to support decision making function in organizations. The sub categorization of MIS as Executive Information Systems and Management Information Systems are just a delineation to differentiate the respective user base on their level of management. This is very important, since the needs of higher level executives and their appetite for details are different from other middle level managers. The main differences in the two types of systems are just apparent in how they present information and knowledge to their audience.

Executive Information Systems

An executive information system (EIS) is a type of management information system that facilitates and supports senior executive information and decision-making needs. It provides easy access to internal and external information relevant to organization goals. It is commonly considered a specialized form of decision support system (DSS)

EIS emphasizes graphical displays and easy-to-use user interfaces. They offer strong reporting and drill-down capabilities. In general, EIS are enterprise-wide DSS that help top-level executives analyze, compare, and highlight trends in important variables so that they can monitor performance and identify opportunities and problems. EIS and data warehousing technologies are converging in the marketplace.

In recent years, the term EIS has lost popularity in favor of business intelligence (with the sub areas of reporting, analytics, and digital dashboards). Wikipedia:- (http://en.wikipedia.org/wiki/Executive_information_system)

The Role of MIS

MIS plays a very critical role in most to all organizations. The data and the Systems of most organizations are like their heart and blood. If I am not afraid, I would say that their relevance to organizations rivals' cash, neck to neck, if not even of higher importance. Relevant data is collected, processed and transformed into pertinent knowledge and information that is appropriately distributed to various end users with the potential to enhance their decision making. Such areas as:
- Query Systems
- Analysis Systems
- Modeling Systems
- Decision Support Systems
- Strategic Planning
- Management Control

- Operational Control
- Transaction Processing etc

All these systems and processes and more depending on the organization's needs comes under the MIS umbrella, hence it encompasses several functional and operational sub-systems. Many organizations will paralyze if their MIS systems break down. It is therefore a very essential pieces of any modern organization, irrespective of their industry. It is even so for Healthcare organizations.

Accountable Care Organizations

"Proponents of accountable-care organizations (ACOs) – consortia of hospitals and physicians that take responsibility for the cost and quality of care – assert that ACOs have the potential to improve patient health while reducing the waste in the healthcare system. But, for the fledgling ACOs to gain traction and begin to achieve that potential, they must build a new kind of technological infrastructure and fundamentally change the way that care is delivered. The optimal ACO infrastructure should be designed to accommodate:

- Consumption of data across disparate clinical and administrative applications and data sources
- Health information exchange across the ACO, regardless of each participant's stage of

Technology adoption
- Core components of an interoperable data exchange, including a Master Patient Index (MPI), a Record Locator Service (RLS), and a patient registry
- Automation tools that provide population health management data and alerts
- Analytics to make data actionable and to evaluate and improve organizational performance" (AT&T Corporation)

The gem in AT&T's proposal of the future of Healthcare IT is kind of engrained in Business Intelligence and Analytics. This combination holds a lot of promise due to the magnitude of data being proliferated out there in the Healthcare Systems. As the saying goes, Data is cheap these days but getting meaning out of it is not. Even better, preventing it in the most appropriate form to the right audience is everything. Function and form are everything, and are essentially equally important, hence BI and Analytics.

"Integrating advanced analytics for Big Data with Business Intelligence Systems is therefore a step towards gaining full return on investments. Advanced Analytics and BI can be highly complementary. Advanced Analytics can provide the deeper, exploratory perspective on the data, while BI systems provide a more structured user experience." (TDWI)

Business Intelligence and Analytics

"Business intelligence (BI) is an umbrella term that includes the applications, infrastructure and tools, and best practices that enable access to and analysis of information to improve and optimize decisions and performance". (Gartner)

"Analytics -- The scientific process of transforming data into insight for making better decisions." (INFORM)

BI and Analytics Vs Decision Support Systems

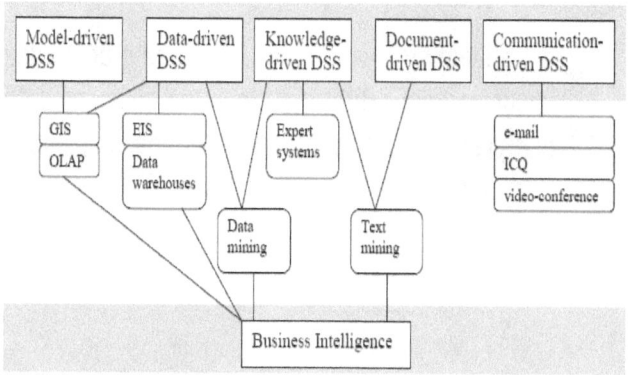

Figure 4

Components of BI and DSS (Hana Kopackova, Et al: University of Pardubice)

Business Intelligence: (BI) is a broad category of applications and technologies for gathering, storing, analyzing, and providing access to data to help enterprise users make better business decisions.

Vs

A decision support system: (DSS) is a computer program application that analyzes business data and presents it so that users can make business decisions more easily.

A brief Historical view of BI and Analytics

In a 1958 article, IBM researcher Hans Peter Luhn used the term business intelligence. He defined intelligence as: "the ability to apprehend the interrelationships of presented facts in such a way as to guide action towards a desired goal."

Business intelligence as it is understood today is said to have evolved from the decision support systems that began in the 1960s and developed throughout the mid-1980s. DSS originated in the computer-aided models created to assist with decision making and planning. From DSS, data warehouses, Executive Information Systems, OLAP and business intelligence came into focus beginning in the late 80s.

In 1989, Howard Dresner (later a Gartner Group analyst) proposed "business intelligence" as an umbrella term to describe "concepts and methods to improve business decision making by using fact-based support systems." It was not until the late 1990s that this usage was widespread.

Business intelligence (BI) today, is a set of theories, methodologies, processes, architectures, and technologies that transform raw data into meaningful and useful information for business purposes. BI can handle large amounts of information to help identify and develop new opportunities. Making use of new opportunities and implementing an effective strategy can provide a competitive market advantage and long-term stability.

BI technologies provide historical, current and predictive views of business operations. Common functions of business

intelligence technologies are reporting, online analytical processing, analytics, data mining, process mining, complex event processing, business performance management, benchmarking, text mining, predictive analytics and prescriptive analytics.
(http://en.wikipedia.org/wiki/Business_intelligence)

Technology Integration

In some deployed business intelligence environments, multiple BI systems – each with their tools, processes and data architectures – can be found across multiple business units and divisions of the Enterprise. These non-integrated BI systems (whether built in-house or acquired) result in high component redundancy, inconsistent knowledge information, proprietary, non-open standard integration interfaces, and highly Maintained point-to-point integration. These ultimately increase the cost of development and prevent the achievement of a single version of truth across the organization.

For business intelligence to deliver on its promises of Real time, zero latency information delivery and closed loop processing, technologies and techniques have emerged. One such evolution is the transformation of traditional BI architectures into service oriented, component-based ones. We believe that Service Oriented Architecture (SOA) technology has great potential for delivering enhanced BI.

Why BI & Analytics in Health Care?

Scott Wanless and Thomas Ludwig in their book, "Business Intelligence and Analytics for Healthcare Organizations, effectively articulated the dying need for Business Intelligence and Analytics in helping to address most of the pressing issues in healthcare today. The major five challenges they cited were as follows:

- Demand Issues
- Resource Shortages
- Compliance requirements
- Financial pressures
- Integration issues

To quote them, "the organization is being pushed and pulled, squeezed and stretched, kicked, thrown, hit and bounced around" by these challenges. The ACO concept, which is tied into their bread and butter, has even exacerbated the challenges, prompting the need for a very well balanced approach that will yield the appropriate clinical and financial remunerations to keep the organizations going in a healthy way. Otherwise their quest to pursue Health and quality of life for others, will infringe enough unsustainable stresses on them, with the potential to cause their extinction.

It may sound gloomy at this point given the challenges out there, yet there is a lot of hope. The current big data revolution, which has triggered a myriad of research and related innovations, in the healthcare industry as well as other industries hold a lot of promise. The tons of data generated everyday in the process of delivering care and their related administrative and operational functions, also contributing, have embedded in them a gem of knowledge and great insights, which can help healthcare practitioners and administrators, make much better decisions. This will ultimately engender more positive outcomes in the areas of need. This eventually will alleviate the apparent pain.

Healthcare Domains with Common Analytical Questions

- "Clinical" Analytical Questions
- "Operational" Analytical Questions
- "Financial" Analytical Questions
- "Administrative" Analytical Questions
- "Public Health" Analytical Questions

BI Competency Center

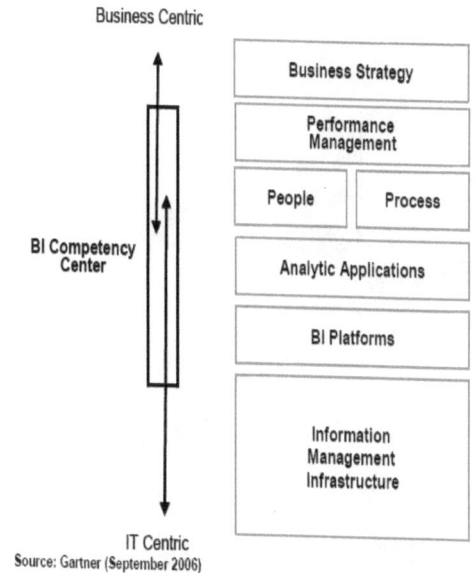

Figure 5

The Basic Health Informatics Theory

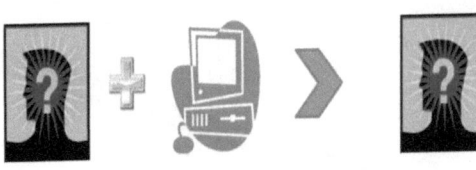

Figure 6

The basic Health Informatics theory is summarized in the above figure. Essentially, it portrays that, the mind and computer aids working together, can help improve the quality and effectiveness of decisions, more so than the relying on the mind alone. Hence, the combination of the mind and computer aids or systems has a greater power in decision making, than the mind by itself. This applies to both clinical and administrative as well as public health and all other healthcare domains of interest.

BI and the Electronic Health Records

Most clinical health care delivery processes as well as research generate a ton of data which provides an excellent environment for a search for useful knowledge and insights. The combination of both structured and unstructured data gashing into healthcare repositories daily provides an excellent opportunity for analytical work in search of formidable insight to aid decision making both in management and also support evidence based medical practice. With Electronic Health Records (EHR) becoming also an involuntary strategic imperative, there is a need to apply data mining and other BI techniques to bring meaning out of them to provide the necessary real time support for evidence based practice for healthcare practitioners, especially physicians. Business Intelligence (BI) has emerged as a formidable technology, which holds a lot of promise in transforming the repository content of EHR in supporting evidence-based practice and improving the quality of healthcare delivery.

The reach of the EHR infrastructure which potentially integrates a greater majority of stakeholders in the Healthcare arena will obviously have a very wide scope of audience. This fluidity amongst the entire pertinent players will even spear head collaborations in research and innovations as well as the general operational nuances of healthcare practice and delivery. The ease of critical information exchange amongst all players in the field, with strict adherence to HIPPA regulations can also be a great "saving" grace. Literally, I mean saving a ton of money by avoiding duplications in diagnostic tests and unnecessary procedures.

BI therefore holds a lot of promise, by unleashing great potential from the myriad of data out there, to support evidence based medicine. Also this will eventually improve healthcare outcomes and quality of life of patients. BI and HER therefore is a good marriage with great recompense.

BI an integrated Summary View of Health Care Information

The end result of BI, which lies in its presentation of useful information to decision makers, does so in providing an integrative summary of views which are easily digestible and synthesized by busy professionals and leaders. Summarizing a tone of data into a simple dashboard with information needed to make a cutting edge or very sensitive decisions with a lot of risk exposures is very ingenious. This simple and fancy look which is presented to the respective stakeholders, holds a lot of mitigating influence on the embedded risk in the respective clinical and administrative decisions.

BI – An Efficiency and Effectiveness Steroid

BI and Analytics infrastructure holds a lot of computational power and speed, which in some situations present useful real time knowledge to healthcare practitioners that make their decisions very effective and efficient. It is therefore a very formidable apparatus of strategic imperative that no organization in the ecosystem can do without eventually. The effectiveness and efficiency factors alone can offset the capital investment that went into its procurement overtime. It is however not even a choice anymore, the way the healthcare practice is heading. Any serious Healthcare organization will either have to get it or be faced out by competitors armed with the edge which the great insights provided by BI and Analytics afford them.

Basic Architecture

- Operational Systems
- Data Repository
- Analytical Applications

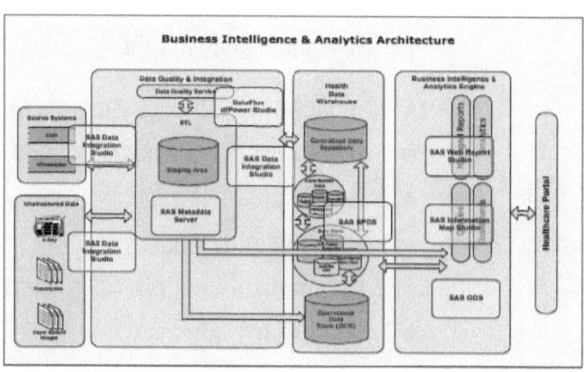

Healthcare Business Intelligence and Analytics Architecture: (SAS)

Figure 7

Targeted Outcomes for BI and Analytics Engagements

- Clinical Success
- Financial Success
- Operational Success
- Enterprise-Wide Success
- Public Health Success

BI – Successes in Health Care

- Reduction in administrative cost
- Discovery of new revenue opportunities
- Supply cost optimization
- Fraud identification
- Detection of cost effective treatments
- Disease management

Interesting Issues

The principal objectives of business intelligence can be summed up as follows:

- To provide a "single version of the truth" across an entire organization.
- To provide a simplified system implementation, deployment and administration
- To deliver strategic, tactical and operational knowledge and actionable insight

Advanced Analytics Adaptation Issues

Though there are a few obstacles for some small and medium size companies primarily on the adaptation of Big Data Analytics, it is growing at a very fast pace. Many companies are reaping numerous benefits from insights gained in advanced analytics using Big Data. Its growing popularity and prominence in the market place, and its numerous promises to many different industries, will trigger the emergence of it becoming a critical strategic imperative for most businesses and organizations. The main catalysts are availability of related technologies, sound business management, and economics.

Obstacles to BI Widespread Adoption

- Lack of resources.
- Complexity of IT systems.
- Future uncertainties & Benefits
- Dissimilar systems posing integration challenges
- Organizational Culture and Politics
- Data quality and Governance
- Lack of Leadership Sponsorship in some cases
- Privacy Laws and Regulations (HIPPA)

Problems or Opportunities

Primarily, the technical challenges in Big Data Analytics and its integration with the BI platform are seen by a minority of organizations as a problem, yet to a vast majority of organization, it is seen as a great innovation with lots of promise and opportunities. A survey conducted by TDWI revealed that only 30% of surveyed organizations saw Big Data Analytics as a problem due to its technical challenges. Yet majority (70%) considered it as a great opportunity.

Other BI Momentum Drivers in the Healthcare Industry

- Evidence Based Management
- Competition and Resource Scarcity
- Smart Customer Base
- Need for More Precision in Decision Making Globally
- A Government Push for EHR:
- High Health Care Payer Expectations for higher Outcomes:

- Legislative Imperative for Safety, Patient Privacy, Operational Efficiency and Higher Outcomes
- Financial incentives for meeting high operational and clinical standard embedded in Current Medicare and Medicaid reimbursement rules which other payers have also adapted

Advanced Business Intelligence at Cardinal Health

In the mid-1990s, Cardinal Health's Medical Products and Services Business Implemented SAP P/3, and built an accompanying data warehouse to handle business reporting. Since that time, use of the data warehouse has diffused widely across the enterprise and the business professionals use widely regularly to solve problems and to take advantage of opportunities.

Besides the Data warehouse, the key components of this advanced BI Environment and Cardinal Health's Data Infrastructure (it's enterprise-wide data model, limited set of tools, and robust support environments and it's information culture (its data-driven decision style, business-led IT decision making, dense social Networks, and pull reporting Structure.

Implementation Options and VENDORS

IMPLEMENTATION OPTIONS	VENDORS IN THE SPACE
ANALYTIC PLATFORM	CARADIGM INTELLIGENCE PLATFORM, HEALTHCARE DATA WORKS, IMB HEALTHCARE DATA MODEL, RECOMBATANT
ANALYTICS SERVICES	EXPLORTS, HUMEDICA, LUMERS, PREMIER ALLIANCE, TRUVEN ANALYTIC SUITE
BEST OF BREED POINT SOLUTIONS	ALTASOFT, CRIMSON SUITE, EPSI, MEDEANALYRICS, MIDAS, OMNICELL, MIDVINITIVE
ELECTRONIC MEDICAL RECORDS	ALL SCRIPT SUNRISE, EPIC CLARITY AND COGITO, McKESSON HORIZON, MEDITECH DATA REPOSITORY, SEIMENS DECISION SUPPORT

Figure 8

Section Conclusion

The proliferation of Business Intelligence and Analytics is not necessarily going to kill Medical Decision Support Systems. However, a well-integrated implementation of MDSS and BI infrastructure, will present a much formidable whole which is even more potent than its parts unilaterally. BI and Analytics has become a very formidable component of Health IT with an acute strategic importance. I believe in spite of the hurdles in its widespread implementation today, the current trends in the healthcare industry's "pains " or explosive challenges will trigger a sense of urgency which will spearhead momentum in its adaptation and rapid proliferation. Ultimately, I believe it will be a saving grace for the industry.

Big Data Applications in Health Care

Technology innovations in the past decade has unleashed tons of useful data which when properly analyzed, will provide useful insights, that expose many healthcare organizations to a myriad of opportunities, to improve clinical outcomes, administrative and operational efficiencies which will lead ultimately, to a much improved bottom line, industry wide. The federal government and other public stakeholders moving toward data and information transparency has also released lots of usable, searchable and actionable data which has greatly improved data liquidity in the industry. These events have pushed the industry to a somewhat tipping point in its adaptation to

Advance analytics using Big Data. This can potentially address lost of issues in the industry, among which are, healthcare variability in quality and escalating cost.

The industry has lagged behind others, primarily because of lack of financial incentives or returns on investments in technology historically. It has however become apparent that, it is the most strategic move any organization can make, if they are really serious about surviving the mountings of issues weighing on them, with financial uncertainties leading.

Other factors that decelerated momentum in Healthcare Organizations' technology adaption are as follows:

- Resistance to change by healthcare professionals afraid of their autonomy in clinical decision making using their judgment
- Uncertainty in returns on investment in technology projects
- Privacy issues that stifles data sharing amongst various stake holders inside and outside the organization
- Lack of integrative approach in business processes internally and externally.

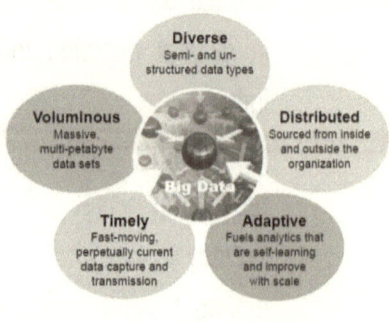

Big Data   Source: McKenzie & Company

Figure 9

The nature of Big Data in healthcare is very diverse and also voluminous. It spans from static to real-time data from many different sources. The humans-system itself comprises of very big data which in a healthcare setting is compartmentalized depending on the department collecting them. This compartmentalization of the data capture point makes it very difficult to ascertain the big picture when it comes to making clinical decisions holistically. An integrative approach to clinical data modeling and processing will make its usefulness in advanced analytics with big data even more beneficial. The very nature of healthcare "big data" and the speed of capture pose a challenge to analyst technically. With the rate at which technology is catching up with the new paradigm, I believe all the nuances will be sorted out in time to unleash its numerous opportunities.

MIT Sloan Management Review & IBM Institute For Business Value: Study Finding

ANALYTICS: The New Path to Value:

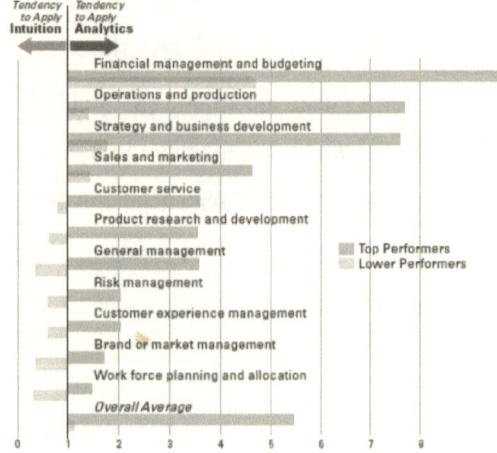

The Tendency for Top – Performing organizing to apply analytic to particular activities across the organizations as compared to lower performers.

Figure 10

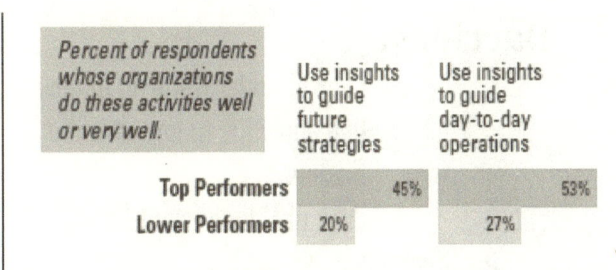

Top performing organizations were twice as likely to use analytics to guide day to day operations and future strategies as lower performers.

Figure 11

> ➢ 60% of Executives Say They "have more information than they can effectively use.
> ➢ The smartest organizations are already capitalizing on increasing information richness and analytics to gain completive advantage.
> ➢ Top performers View analytic as a differentiator.

Barriers:
- Lack of understanding of how to use analytics to improve the Business
- Lack of Management Bandwidth

➤ Strategies:
- Focus on the biggest opportunities first
- Start with Question not Data
- Embed Insight to Drive Actions
- Keep existing Capabilities whiles adding new ones
- Build the Analytics Foundation According to an information Agenda

	ASPIRATIONAL	EXPERIENCED	TRANSFORMED
Motive	• Use analytics to justify actions	• Use analytics to guide actions	• Use analytics to prescribe actions
Functional proficiency	• Financial management and budgeting • Operations and production • Sales and marketing	• All Aspirational functions • Strategy / business development • Customer service • Product research / development	• All Aspirational and Experienced functions • Risk management • Customer experience • Work force planning / allocation • General management • Brand and market management
Business challenges	• Competitive differentiation through innovation • Cost efficiency (primary) • Revenue growth (secondary)	• Competitive differentiation through innovation • Revenue growth (primary) • Cost efficiency (secondary)	• Competitive differentiation through innovation • Revenue growth (primary) • Profitability acquiring / retaining customers (targeted focus)
Key obstacles	• Lack of understanding how to leverage analytics for business value • Executive sponsorship • Culture does not encourage sharing information	• Lack of understanding how to leverage analytics for business value • Skills within line of business • Ownership of data is unclear or governance is ineffective	• Lack of understanding how to leverage analytics for business value • Management bandwidth due to competing priorities • Accessibility of the data
Data management	• Limited ability to capture, aggregate, analyze or share information and insights	• Moderate ability to capture, aggregate and analyze data • Limited ability to share information and insights	• Strong ability to capture, aggregate and analyze data • Effective at sharing information and insights
Analytics in action	• Rarely use rigorous approaches to make decisions • Limited use of insights to guide future strategies or guide day-to-day operations	• Some use of rigorous approaches to make decisions • Growing use of insights to guide future strategies, but still limited use of insights to guide day-to-day operations	• Most use rigorous approaches to make decisions • Almost all use insights to guide future strategies, and most use insights to guide day-to-day operations

[Three Capabilities Level [Apparitional, Experienced & Transformation: Were based on How Respondents rated Their Organization's Analytic Prowes]
Figure 12

Healthcare and Big Data

Healthcare Big Data comes from many different sources with ownership spanning widely across different stakeholder in the ecosystem. Some of these stakeholders are not even in the healthcare industry. In spite of the diversity in data sources and ownership, the potential of big data analytics can only be fully harnessed with an adaptation of an integrative approach to data collection and sharing, among all the dissimilar organization, with varying perspectives and interests.

This alone posed a potential hurdle which needs to be very tactfully navigated due to the apparent political nature of most organization, with their inherent power plays.

Diplomacy therefore is "key" in negotiating such deals.

An Example of BI Implementation in Education: Penn State

Introduction

"The goal of the Business Intelligence initiative was to assess Penn State's current information needs and then to work cooperatively with the University Community to plan, design, develop and implement an infrastructure that would transform administrative data into information and that will make the right information available to the right Penn State stakeholder at the right time and in the right delivery media.

To achieve that we took a three step approach, this included requirements analysis, strategy definition and implementation planning.

In addition, the Business Intelligence Advisory Committee was formed. The main role of the Business Intelligence Advisory Committee was to provide advice throughout the requirements analysis, strategy definition and implementation planning phases of the Business Intelligence Initiative.

The Committee includes representation from a large cross-section of information users....

Findings

The requirement analysis phase included a review of the current Penn State information management environment as well as one-on-one interviews with a comprehensive cross-section of information users, at various management and responsibility levels, covering all major Penn State areas. The focus of the interviews was to understand how people use the information currently available to them and to gauge what the key Penn State information needs are.

In addition, the Business Intelligence Advisory Committee worked extensively on reviewing and further defining both who are the users of information at Penn State as well as what the most pressing information needs are.

Throughout the interview process it was apparent that even though some of the existing information systems, like the Data Warehouse or the Strategic Information Management System (SIMS), are considered extremely valuable and widely used by both academic and academic-support units, those systems were not meeting all existing information needs. Information is not easily available to all Penn State constituencies and significant number of academic leaders, and administrators have very limited access to information.

Significantly, there is a widespread need for improved access to information on both students and overall teaching and learning activities. Reasons for needing this information are tied to improving the ability to make better day to day and long term decisions about how to reach and serve students as well as improving organizational efficiency.

Reasons pointed out during the interview process include understanding learning outcomes, improving student retention, understanding faculty workload, and identifying under-enrolled courses, among others.

A changing operational environment and increased demand and pressure for accountability coming from public policy makers as well as the educational community, have triggered extensive new information needs that the existing information systems do not fully support. Accountability pressures explicitly demand that academic institutions be able to directly link academic performance data and outcome data. Penn State's current information systems do not support this analysis both because the required data are collected and stored in disconnected silos and because data are simply not collected and not available.

Furthermore, responsibilities, decision-making, and accountability regarding data and information are spread across a number of units with no well defined coordination mechanisms. This situation fosters an environment of inconsistent data management policies, and inconsistent and fragmented security.

Strategic Vision for Business Intelligence at Penn State

Given the current operational environment, the push on academic and non-academic units to do more with less will continue to grow. Decision making and planning will increasingly become more cross functional and interdependent.

In addition, regulatory and accountability pressures will continue to expand. For academic and academic-support units to continue to function effectively and efficiently, it is essential that Penn State moves towards a university-wide approach to data management. Data should be looked at as a common asset that can be made into information and knowledge to support effective decision making across all of Penn State. The underlying concept behind the proposed strategic vision is the concept of Penn

State data as a valuable asset that is commonly owned by the university community. Penn State data should be looked at not as a collection of independent fragments but as a flow of interdependent events that provide maximum value only when viewed as a whole.

Strategically, Penn State should move towards providing its information users - staff, faculty, researchers and administrators, among others- with access to a unified and integrated view of Penn State's core data, meaning university-wide data that are needed by a large number of Penn State constituencies and are core to the Penn State mission. This integrated and unified data view will need to be secure, accurate, timely, consistent, intuitive, and easy to obtain so that information users are better able to assess their needs, set priorities, understand the impact of change and thus fulfill their responsibilities more efficiently.

One example of a unified and integrated view of data is the student longitudinal view, which would provide a record of the students' interactions with Penn State from the time when they become a prospect, throughout their interactions as alumni. The student longitudinal view would allow Penn State to have a better understanding of learning outcomes as well as make better day to day and long term decisions about how to reach and serve students.

Key Recommendations

Our key recommendation is that Penn State moves beyond traditional data repositories and from only focusing on data and information reporting for operational purposes towards managing information as a strategic Penn State asset that can be used to provide insight into the institution as a whole.

This recommendation includes three different dimensions:

• Governance and Policy - Orchestration of people, process and technology as to allow Penn State to manage data as an Institution Asset;

• Organizational Structures - Central unit, within Administrative Information Services, that will support the proposed infrastructure and lead effort to implement a university-wide view of data and information;

• Software, Hardware and Data Infrastructure - Centrally supported, within Administrative Information Services, Institution Insight infrastructure.

Information as a Strategic Asset

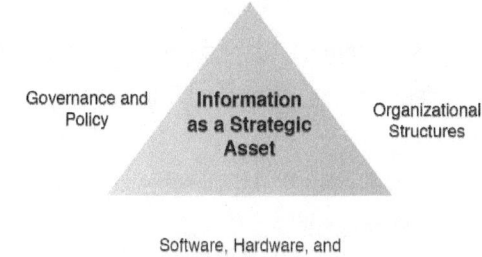

Figure 13

Governance and Policy

The purpose of Governance and Policy is to define and implement mechanisms that ensure the accuracy, integrity, accessibility and security of information across Penn State. These mechanisms will consist of a collection of processes, standards, policies and technologies that will allow Penn Sate manage and use information as a strategic asset.

Among others, Governance and Policy will include initiatives to:

• Further define which data should be considered core Penn State data;

• Review data stewardship model and processes;

• Review data security and privacy models;

• Create a consensus on data policies as well as data definitions for core Penn State attributes.

• Define data quality and integrity standards.

Software, Hardware and Data - the Institution Insight System

The Institution Insight System will consist of a well-integrated arrangement of data repositories, software and hardware components. This system will have the ability to integrate data from a broad spectrum of university information systems and data repositories, and will have the capability to make information available through a multitude of channels.

The Institution Insight System technical infrastructure should be hosted and supported centrally but should be available to all Penn State constituencies to make their data and information available to information users. This system will eventually become the point of entry for the majority of data access and analysis at Penn State......

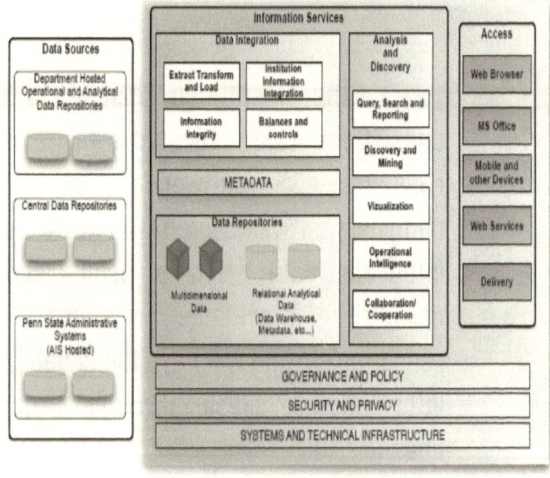

Figure 14

Penn State Institution Insight System:
(SYSTEMS AND TECHNICAL INFRASTRUCTURE)

Furthermore, the Institution Insight System will enable the creation of a unified and integrated view of Penn State's core data. These

data might eventually span the majority of Penn State's academic and academic-support processes. Some of the processes requested by the users include:
- Teaching and learning;
- Enrollment Management;
- Research and scholarship;
- Financial planning and budgeting;
- Faculty recruitment, development and retention;
- Alumni and university relations and management;
- Staff recruitment, development and retention.

Organizational Structures

The successful implementation of the Business Intelligence strategic vision depends upon the existence of organization structures that will support the proposed central infrastructure and university-wide view of data and information.

The Business Intelligence unit will be accountable to the overall Penn State community of information users and will be ultimately responsible for ensuring that the Institution Insight System meets their needs. This organization will work based on the priorities established by the Data Management Council and will take a university-wide perspective on data and information delivery with a focus on core university objectives. Among other things, this organization will develop, implement and manage the Institution Insight System technical infrastructure as well as lead and partially staff the university-wide effort to create the integrated and unified view of Penn State Data....

Moving Forward

Given the information needs expressed by users the first priority of the Institution Insight System should be the establishment of an integrated and unified view of the data and information underlying student and overall teaching and learning activities related processes.

Given the scope and complexity of the Institution Insight System, its successful implementation will require continued close partnership of functional and technical personnel, drawing skills and participation from across a variety of Penn State units.

The implementation must be divided into a series of smaller, manageable iterations. An iterative approach will start creating value-added for the users within a shorter time-frame and will allow the project team to refine their methods and techniques with each iteration. Iterative implementations are a proven technique for mitigating the risk associated with large Business Intelligence deployments.

The first iteration will establish the required organization structure and pilot the Institution Insight System information access and delivery technical infrastructure. Following iterations will add to the existing content as well as continue to finetune the overall infrastructure...." [Penn State University]

Part II

MANAGING HEALTHCARE WITH DATA & RELATED BENEFITS

Introduction

Big Data Analytics is a new buzz word in technology which has proven itself in many industries to be a formidable tool in addressing lots of issues of importance with relatively better precision. The advent of Web 2 technologies and many others in recent times has made available tons of important business related data. To generate meaning out of this raw data, it will need to be diligently analyzed.

Upon analysis, very important patterns and insights are revealed, which are critical to business decision making, most especially in highly unstructured ones with enough crippling potential uncertainties.

These business insights often improve current business operations, as well as unleash a lot of potential opportunities in the market place. Most often, it also enhances the discovery of strategic innovative initiatives pertinent to the success of organizations. Overall is has been a strategic imperative in providing innovative companies a huge competitive edge. It's adaptation in the Healthcare industry however has not been at par with other industries. The tardiness of the healthcare industry in the adaptation of Big Data analytics however, has some historical connotations pertaining to the industry's culture in general. Healthcare organizations generally rank complex technology initiative at the low end of their priority spectrum, due to the haziness in quantifying their return on investment among other factors. The industry at the moment is facing numerous challenges.

Potentially, it is even over exposed to a financial catastrophe due to the country's apparent demographic composition. The dominant aging population and the potential surge due to the Baby Boomers is a matter of great concern. It poses enough threat, which can cripple the system financially if not addressed well in advance. A pre-emptive move to avert the catastrophe is therefore very necessary to help save the country from it escalating fiscal economic woes. This potential healthcare sector's escalating financial stress can very adversely affect the nation's already dismal budget deficit issue that is looming on us. As an antidote to leaving such a big problem to posterity and our ailing parents and grandparents, Big Data Analytics holds a lot of promise, and this paper will attempt to illustrate why.

Business Intelligence and Analytics

"Business intelligence (BI) is an umbrella term that includes the applications, infrastructure and tools, and best practices that enable access to and analysis of information to improve and optimize decisions and performance". (Gartner)

"Analytics — The scientific process of transforming data into insight for making better decisions."
(INFORM)

A Brief Historical Perspective

In a 1958 article, IBM researcher Hans Peter Luhn used the term business intelligence. He defined intelligence as: "the ability to apprehend the interrelationships of presented facts in such a way as to guide action towards a desired goal." Business intelligence as it is understood today is said to have evolved from the decision support systems that began in the 1960s and developed throughout the mid-1980s. DSS originated in the computer-aided models created to assist with decision making and planning. From DSS, data warehouses, Executive Information Systems, OLAP and business intelligence came into focus beginning in the late 80s. In 1989, Howard Dresner (later a Gartner Group analyst) proposed "business intelligence" as an umbrella term to describe "concepts and methods to improve business decision making by using fact-based support systems."

It was not until the late 1990s that this usage was widespread. Business intelligence (BI) today, is a set of theories, methodologies, processes, architectures, and technologies that transform raw data into meaningful and useful information for business purposes. BI can handle large amounts of information to help identify and develop new opportunities. Making use of new opportunities and implementing an effective strategy can provide a competitive market advantage and long-term stability.

BI technologies provide historical, current and predictive views of business operations. Common functions of business intelligence technologies are reporting, online analytical processing, analytics, data mining, process mining, complex event processing, business performance management, benchmarking, text mining, predictive analytics and prescriptive analytics. (http://en.wikipedia.org/wiki/Business intelligence)

Challenges facing the Healthcare Space
- Increased Demand for Services
- Resource Shortage
- Compliance Requirements
- Financial Pressures and Stresses on the System
- Vertical and Horizontal Integration

Healthcare Domains with Common Analytical Questions
- "Clinical" Analytical Questions
- "Operational" Analytical Questions
- "Financial" Analytical Questions
- "Administrative" Analytical Questions
- "Public Health" Analytical Questions

Basic Architecture

- Operational Systems
- Data Repository
    - Analytical Applications

Targeted Outcomes for BI and Analytics Engagements

- ✓ Clinical Success
- ✓ Financial Success
- ✓ Operational Success
- ✓ Enterprise-Wide Success
- ✓ Public Health Success

So far it can be safely concluded that Business Intelligence and Analytics falls right in the Informatics domain of disciplines, and in fact holds a lot of promise now and in the future. It is indeed a very formidable tool which can go a long way in helping to address the myriad of healthcare woes in our current system.

BI AND BIG DATA: AN INTEGRATED VIEW

According to TDWI, I quote: "Big data is growing fast as organizations devote technology resources to tapping the terabytes (if not petabytes) of data flowing into their organizations and externally in social media data and other sources. What does this all mean for business intelligence (BI) users and systems? With all the attention on advanced analytics for big data, what's the play for BI? Integrating advanced analytics for big data with BI systems is an important step toward gaining full return on investment. Advanced analytics and BI can be highly complementary; advanced analytics can provide the deeper, exploratory perspective on the data, while BI systems provide a more structured user experience. BI systems' richness in dashboard visualization, reporting, performance management metrics and more can be vital to making advanced analytics actionable". (TDWI)

BI – BIG DATA ANALYTICS: ADVANCED ANALYTICS

[Some Common Definitions Advanced Analytics: A discovery Mission]

Advanced Analytics is a collection of related techniques, process and tools, which usually include; predictive analytics, data mining, statistical analysis, and complex SQL. It also includes, data visualization, artificial intelligence, natural language processing and database capabilities that support analytics. (eg. MapReduce, in-database analytics, in-memory databases, columnar data stores etc.

The main objective of advanced analytics is to sift through massive amount of variety of data to identify patterns and business facts which are yet to be discovered by either the industry or the company. These facts and insights support their strategic moves or solve major crippling problems, or sometimes improve operational efficiencies, or customer satisfaction. Ultimately these tend to improve sales and increase revenue and profits. Big data discoveries mixed with historical data from the data warehouse, leads to a metric, report, analytic tools, or some other BI products to support decision making in the company. Advanced analytics can be enabled by different type of analytic tools, including SQL based queries, data mining, statistical analysis, fact clustering, data visualization, natural language processing, text analytics, artificial intelligence and a wide arsenal of tools which requires a savvy professional to access the needs of a particular organization.

Big Data Analytics

Big Data Analytics is where advanced analytics tools and techniques are used to operate on Big Data, to achieve the ends as has already been addressed previously in this document.

Interesting Adaptation Issues

Though there are a few obstacles for some small and medium size companies primarily on the adaptation of Big Data Analytics, it is growing at a very fast pace. Many companies are reaping numerous benefits from insights gained in advanced analytics using Big Data. Its growing popularity and prominence in the market place, and its numerous promises to many different industries, will trigger the emergence of it becoming a critical strategic imperative for most businesses and organizations. The main catalysts are availability of related technologies, sound business management, and economics.

Obstacles to Big Data Analytics Widespread Adoption

The above figure highlights some of the critical factors that hamper the smooth growth of this innovative technology which holds such great promises. In spite of all these challenges, I believe that the current momentum will continue if not accelerate. It is going to be so, because the technology is improving very fast and the timing is also right with favorable industry environmental factors.

Problems or Opportunities

Primarily, the technical challenges in Big Data Analytics and its integration with the BI platform are seen by a minority of organizations as a problem, yet to a vast majority of organization, it is seen as a great innovation with lots of promise and opportunities. A survey conducted by TDWI revealed that only 30% of surveyed organizations saw Big Data Analytics as a problem due to its technical challenges. Yet majority (70%) considered it as a great opportunity.

Big Data Applications In Healthcare

Technology innovations in the past decade has unleashed tons of useful data which when properly analyzed, will provide useful insights, that exposes many healthcare organizations to a myriad of opportunities, to improve clinical outcomes, administrative and operational efficiencies which will lead ultimately, to a much improved bottom line, industry wide.

The federal government and other public stakeholders moving toward data and information transparency has also released lots of usable, searchable and actionable data which has greatly improved data liquidity in the industry. These events have pushed the industry to a somewhat tipping point in its adaptation to

Advanced analytics using Big Data. This can potentially address lots of issues in the industry, among which are, healthcare variability in quality and escalating cost. The industry has lagged behind others, primarily because of lack of financial incentive or return on investments in technology historically. It has however become apparent that, it is the most strategic move any organization can make, if they are really serious about surviving the mountings of issues weighing on them, with financial uncertainties leading. Other factors that decelerated momentum in Healthcare Organizations' technology adaption are as follows:

- Resistance to change by healthcare professionals afraid of their autonomy in clinical decision making using their judgment
- Uncertainty in return on investment in technology projects

- Privacy issues that stifles data sharing amongst various stakeholders inside and outside the organization
- Lack of integrative approach in business processes internally and externally.

    The nature of Big Data in healthcare is very diverse and also voluminous. It spans from static to real-time data from many different sources. The humans-system itself comprises of very big data which in a healthcare setting is compartmentalized making it very difficult to ascertain the big picture when it comes to making clinical decisions holistically. An integrative approach to clinical data modeling and processing will make its usefulness in advanced analytics with big data even more beneficial. The very nature of healthcare "big data" and the speed of capture pose a challenge to analyst technically. With the rate at which technology is catching up with the new paradigm, I believe all the nuances will be sorted out in time to unleash its numerous opportunities.

Health Care and Big Data

Healthcare Big Data comes from many different sources with ownership spanning widely across different stakeholders in the ecosystem. Some of these stakeholders are not even in the healthcare industry. In spite of the diversity in data sources and ownership, the potential of big data analytics can only be fully harnessed with an adaptation of an integrative approach to data collection and sharing, among all the dissimilar organization, with varying perspectives and interests.

This alone posed a potential hurdle which needs to be very tactfully navigated due to the apparent political nature of most organization, with their inherent power plays.

Diplomacy therefore is "key" in negotiating such deals. Besides the nuances of dealing with the different interest groups with varying priorities, there are some real technical and business challenges that decelerate the momentum of Big Data Analytics in healthcare organizations is a chart by Mackenzie and Company which highlights some of the human, technical and business hurdles and challenges that needs to be addressed to accelerate its natural pace. Challenging as it may seem as explained in the previous paragraph, the industry cannot simply afford to miss this opportunity. They are compelled to jump on the band wagon, and ride diligently to harness its invaluable potential and opportunities.

Competitive imperatives, liquidity of data, technological advancements, and government initiatives and incentive structures have pushed the industry to a tipping edge. The chart below shows some of the industry wide paradigm shifts that have propelled the need for advanced analytics to enhance both clinical operational and administrative outcomes. This is very critical to almost all healthcare organizations since it directly or indirectly affects their bottom line, (Profits) and their very ability to compete and exist. The new paradigm shift has chanced how the industry perceives value which affects their income potential.

The value pathways as described below shows which outcomes are most important to their bottom line. It is therefore apparent that customer satisfaction, operational and clinical outcomes has become paramount and essential to the survival of most Healthcare organizations. To achieve these ends with some level of precision, and avoid pitfalls that engender wasteful spending, organizations need lots of insight and decision support aids to help decision makers avoid costly and preventable mistakes.

Potential Impact of Big Data on the Health Care System

In brief, according to McKenzie & Company, the US healthcare system can enjoy a savings of 300 to 450 Billion dollars over time, which can relieve the industry of its looming financial stresses. These results are achievable, if advanced analytics is properly implemented and expected outcomes, diligently managed. The bottom line benefit however goes beyond the financial incentives. The improvement in the quality of life of our population can also translate into high productivity, which ultimately will piggy bag on the financial gains due to the cost containment factor and therefore creates a healthy economy.

Other Big Data Momentum Drivers in the Healthcare Industry

- Evidence Based Management
- Competition and Resource Scarcity
- Smart Customer Base
- Need for More Precision in Decision Making Globally
- A Government Push for EHR:
- High Health Care Payer Expectations for Higher

Outcomes:

- Legislative Imperative for Safety, Patient Privacy, Operational Efficiency and Higher Outcomes
- Financial incentives for meeting high operational and clinical standards embedded in Current Medicare and Medicaid Reimbursement rules which other payers have also adopted

Some Industry Wide Imperatives

- Establishing a common ground for data governance and usability
- Shifting the collective mind-set about patient data to share, with protection, rather than protect
- Invest in the capabilities of all the players that will share and work with data:

  ➢ Data Analysis
  ➢ Data Management
  ➢ Systems Management

Section Conclusion

With the evidence provided in this section, it is very apparent that the current healthcare environmental nuances, coupled with the paradigm shifts in their value propositions, and insurmountable pressure on the entire system, driven by demand, resource and financial scarcity, legislative imperatives among others, leave very little room for apathy. It is therefore a strategic imperative not only for the industry, but the country as a whole, because the US government is the largest payer in the healthcare system. Its share of responsibility is potentially going to balloon due to the current demographic composition of the country pertaining to population.

The aging baby boomer population in the country poses a very big financial risk to its social programs designed to alleviate human pain and suffering. Beyond our borders, the population composition is not that different in many countries, and therefore our current potential threat is not an isolated situation. It is very important that the global community rallies around this issue and find an innovative solution to avert the crisis. At the moment, Big Data Analytics seems to be one of the best tools available, with the technical and economic feasibility to address the potential pandemonium of such global magnitude.

PART III

IMPLEMENTATION EXAMPLES & CHALLENGES - [UK]

[Michael Karpf, MD: Executive Vice President for Health Affairs: UK HealthCare, University of Kentucky UK: - Information Technology Strategic Plan. An enterprise wide Initiative to solidify the future 2012 Source: [UK HEALTHCARE: MAGAZINE]]

UK HealthCare physician faculty and dedicated staff lead the advanced specialty care in the region and recognize the critical role information technology (IT) plays in achieving our medical and business strategies. Additionally, IT will be a fundamental organizer in relationship development and making improvements to care delivery. Our dedicated teams of clinicians, operations, finance and IT specialists are in pursuit of a single patient record to be distributed across our health care enterprise. Eventually, this record will be shared with providers across the Commonwealth and beyond to ensure they have current information while caring for members of our community.

This single record will contain valuable data which can be used as a strategic asset to improve UK HealthCare. Over the last decade, we have made significant investments and have laid the foundation for our ever-increasing data and information needs in this era of health care reform. Investments in information technology (IT) will enable UK HealthCare to improve patient care, enhance communication with providers, adhere to regulations and operate profitably. The overarching goal is to have a single patient record that can be shared across the health care enterprise to improve the quality of care we provide to our patients. Information technology will be a fundamental organizer in relationship development and making improvements to care delivery. Therefore, UK HealthCare has invested heavily in information technology.

UK HealthCare Information Technology will partner more closely with our medical and business functions in the years ahead. We will dedicate ourselves to building upon our strong momentum and living our vision. The main area of investment in IT has included the automation of the inpatient medical record. Currently, UK HealthCare's electronic health record (EHR) includes computerized physician order entry (CPOE), electronic medication administration and online nursing documentation. Additionally, information systems have been implemented in the majority of UK HealthCare's clinical areas, such as surgery, the emergency department, laboratories, radiology imaging and pharmacy. Additionally, major IT Investments have been made to support UK HealthCare's growth and system integration strategies. Several multi-years IT projects were completed to provide state-of-the-art information systems in both the new pavilion at UK Albert B.

Upcoming IT efforts in the inpatient setting will include the expansion of electronic physician documentation, the optimization of currently installed systems and improved analytics capabilities. These actions will continue to enhance our abilities to better serve patients in the inpatient settings, as well as position us for further system development. Continued investments in health care IT for the ambulatory settings are also being pursued. Implementing an electronic medical record in the ambulatory clinics is a key component to our strategies. These investments will ensure accurate and complete patient information from all of our care settings is available to providers at any time and from any place. Following the success of the physician portal, UK HealthCare will pursue development of a secure patient portal. The ability to look up education will be part of this functionality.

UK HealthCare will continue to pursue future meaningful use components, including Exchange (KHIE). Major implementations in our registration, admission, scheduling and billing information IT investment plan. Operational effectiveness and efficiency.

IT will play a critical role in the organization's plans to develop closer working relationships and collaborations with community hospitals and providers. In order to operate as a more structured system, IT must be leveraged to provide information about the patient to all of the patient's caregivers no matter where a provider is located within the system.

[EHR IMPLEMENTATION PROGRESSION IN UK – FROM 2008 & EARLIER]

- Inpatient EMR/CPOE
- Surgery Info System
- Lab
- Radiology
- Registration
- Scheduling
- Billing
- Financial Decision Support
- Acute & Critical Care
- Clinical Documentation
- PACS
- HIMS/Medical Records
- Cardiology
- eMAR

[EHR IMPLEMENTATION PROGRESSION IN UK – FROM 2009 & 2010]

- Document Image Scanning
- Patient Access Center
- EMR in ED
- Inpatient Pharmacy
- Bed Management
- Physician Documentation
- Good Samaritan Hospital Integration
- New Patient Care Facility - ED
- Lab Specimen Collection
- Analytics
- Outpatient Pharmacy
- Risk Management
- Central Telemetry
- Rx Writer
- Physician Portal

[EHR IMPLEMENTATION PROGRESSION IN UK – FROM 2011 & 2012]

- New Patient Care Facility - Inpatient/ICU
- Ambulatory EMR Selection
- Georgetown Clinic EMR
- Health Information Exchange
- New Patient Care Facility - OR
- New Patient Care Facility - Data Center
- Encryption
- Inpatient EMR Meaningful Use Upgrade
- Meaningful Use Eligible
- Hospital Stage 1 Attestation
- Facility Boards

[The complexity of developing an electronic medical record is illustrated. UK HealthCare has already implemented a majority of the components and is now actively pursuing the most complex components such as the patient health record, health information exchange and data warehouse. UK HealthCare]

What Revenue Cycle is Doing

1. Health care payments, reform & regulatory compliance
    - ✓ ICD-10
    - ✓ Provider-based clinics
    - ✓ Payor contracting
    - ✓ Governmental payor cost reporting
    - ✓ Bundling payments
    - ✓ Accountable care organization
    - ✓ Quality reporting systems
    - ✓ Electronic facsimile solution
    - ✓ American Recovery & Reinvestment Act
    - ✓ Health information management

2. Quality initiatives & compliance
    - ✓ Master patient index optimization
    - ✓ Consolidation of complete record

- ✓ Handheld dictation devices
- ✓ Compliance tracking optimization
- ✓ Quality module software
- ✓ Electronic health record
- ✓ Chart abstracting & scanning
- ✓ Electronic physician query
- ✓ Physician clinical documentation
- ✓ Computer-assisted coding

3. Account receivables management
    - ✓ Integrate Central Kentucky Management Services functions
    - ✓ Enterprise accounts receivable solution
    - ✓ Patient access portal
    - ✓ Propensity-to-pay optimization
    - ✓ Pricing estimator optimization
    - ✓ Improve charge master compliance
    - ✓ Reduce initial claim rejection
    - ✓ Eliminate paper charge process

- ✓ Enterprise denial management
- ✓ Third-party financing

How IT Can Help

1. Health care payments, reform & regulatory compliance
   - ✓ ICD-10 implementation
   - ✓ Provider-based clinics
   - ✓ Payor modeling
   - ✓ Governmental payor cost report
   - ✓ Accountable Care Organization
   - ✓ Quality reporting systems
   - ✓ Electronic facsimile
   - ✓ American Recovery & Reinvestment Act metric solutions
   - ✓ Health information management

2. Quality initiatives & compliance
   - ✓ Master patient index maintenance

- ✓ Electronic record optimization
- ✓ Handheld dictation device
- ✓ Compliance tracking
- ✓ Quality module software
- ✓ Physician clinical documentation
- ✓ Computer-assisted coding
- ✓ Chart scanning and abstraction for AEHR

3. Account receivables management
   - ✓ Central Kentucky Management Services system
   - ✓ Enterprise accounts receivable
   - ✓ Patient access portal
   - ✓ Charge master optimization
   - ✓ Propensity-to-pay optimization
   - ✓ Pricing estimator optimization
   - ✓ Eliminate paper charging
   - ✓ Enterprise denial management

What Strategic Planning is Doing
1. Decision support
    - ✓ Reliable and high-quality data
    - ✓ Advanced electronic tools for decision support
    - ✓ External reporting for UK HealthCare data
    - ✓ Assessment and acquisition of a new decision support system
2. Growth & Outreach
    - ✓ Partnerships with external providers and facilities
        - Remote clinical management of patients
        - Telemedicine clinical application
        - Telemedicine enhanced Communication
        - Continuing education
        - Physician portal

- ✓ Enabling internal providers in remote outreach locations

How IT Can Help

1. Decision support
    - ✓ Decision-support application delivery
    - ✓ Data stewardship and retention of reliable data

2. Growth & outreach
    - ✓ Physician portal
    - ✓ Telemedicine
    - ✓ Remote application delivery at outreach sites

Initiatives

What Supply Chain is Doing
1. Warehouse automation
    - ✓ Systems, Applications and Products (SAP) bar-coding solution
    - ✓ Inventory management
    - ✓ Return rate reduction
2. Pick list automation
    - ✓ Standardization
3. PYXIS
    - ✓ Hospital implementation
4. Decision-support system
    - ✓ University HealthSystem Consortium (UHC) tool
5. Standardization
    - ✓ Case-specific physician preferences

- ✓ Ekahau wireless real-time location system (RTLS)

How IT Can Help

1. Warehouse automation
    - ✓ Systems, Applications and Products (SAP) bar-coding solution
    - ✓ Inventory management system
2. Pick list automation
    - ✓ Carousel implementations
    - ✓ Automation optimization
3. PYXIS
    - ✓ Hospital implementation
4. Decision-support system
    - ✓ Tools
    - ✓ Database
5. Standardization
    - ✓ Ekahau optimization

The following governance subcommittees have been established, or are in the process of being established, to assist with specific themes and challenges:

- ✓ Project request prioritization
- ✓ Data warehouse
- ✓ Infrastructure and security
- ✓ Service request prioritization

Key Attributes of a World-Class IT Organization:

[IT's vision is to "Build a World-Class IT Function to Transform Health Care." We adopted an industry best practices framework with the following components:]

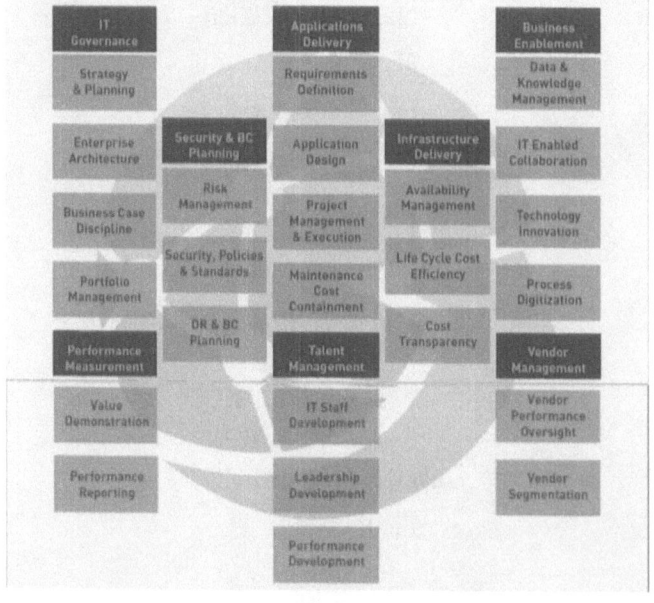

Source: Corporate Executive Board, Key Attributes of the World-Class Information Technology Organization. [UK HealthCare]

Figure 15

Ambulatory Services Strategy:

1. Transition of care (creating an integrated patient experience)
2. Space optimization
3. Access
4. Ambulatory services standardization

Input provided by:
Jonathan Curtright
Marc Randall, MD

Behavioral Health Strategy:

1. Clinical documentation
2. Patient units
3. Best practices

Input provided by:
Darlene Spalding

Cardiology Strategy:

1. Electrophysiology and catheterization Lab
2. Imaging
3. Outreach
4. Inpatient services
5. Clinic
6. Cardiac rehabilitation
7. Cardiovascular research
8. Education
9. Administration

Input provided by:

Justin Campbell
Rick McClure, MD
Susan Smyth, MD, PhD
Vincent Sorrell, MD

Chief Medical Information Officer Strategy

1. Optimization of clinical systems
2. Centralized data warehouse
3. Outreach and growth
4. IT recognition

Input provided by:

Carol Steltenkamp, MD

Clinical Network Strategy

Affiliate network
1. Outreach clinics network
2. Community division network
3. Network access and reporting

Input provided by:

Joe Claypool

Karen Riggs

Clinical Performance Strategy

1. High-quality care, patient safety & service
2. Providing the most efficient care
3. Standardized care
4. Continuum of care focus

Input provided by:

Paul DePriest, MD
Carol Steltenkamp, MD

College of Medicine Strategy

1. Continuing education central function
2. Enterprise research storage
Input provided by:
Fred de Beer, MD

Compliance Strategy

　　1. Privacy & security
　　2. Research
　　3. Billing
　　4. Conflict of interest

Input provided by:

　　Andrew Hill
　　Brett Short

Critical Care Strategy

　　1. High-quality care & patient safety
　　2. Providing most efficient care
　　3. Data-based decision-making
　　4. Improve outcomes
　　Input provided by:
　　Pam Branson
　　Kathleen Kopser

Scott Morehead, MD

Development Strategy

1. Enterprise & College of Medicine fundraising activities
2. Fundraising audiences & approaches

Input provided by:
Vickie Myers
Brad Smetanko

Emergency Department Strategy

1. High-quality care & patient safety
2. Providing most efficient care
3. Data-based decision-making
4. Improved outcomes
5. Community integration

Input provided by:

Penne Allison

External Affairs Strategy

1. Central Web function
2. Access Center
3. Contracts, vendor relationships
4. Health care reform
5. Portfolio Management Office optimization
6. Employee linkages
7. Affiliations

Input provided by:

Mark Birdwhistell
Rob Edwards

Finance Hospital Strategy

1. Hospital accounting

2. Long-term capital forecasting
3. Capital portfolio management

Input provided by:

Byron Gabbard
Jay Sial

Financial Planning Strategy

1. Maintain leading-edge financial systems
2. Better utilize campus applications

Input provided by: Teresa Centers

Good Samaritan Strategy

1. Community hospital system growth
2. Enterprise service optimization
3. Infrastructure optimization and expansion

Input provided by:

Ann Smith
Darlene Spalding

Graduate Medical Education Strategy

1. Informatics as a core competency in medical education
2. Innovations in medical education
3. Supporting a culture of safety
4. Improved communication strategies

Input provided by

Susan McDowell, MD

Departments & Functional Areas

1. Markey Cancer Center Strategy
2. Neurosciences Strategy
3. Nursing Strategy

4. Obstetrics Strategy
5. Perioperative Services Strategy
6. Pharmacy Strategy
7. Radiation Medicine Strategy
8. Radiology Strategy
9. Trauma
10. Surgry Strategy

Revenue Cycle Strategy

1. Health care payments, reform & regulatory compliance
2. Quality initiatives & compliance
3. Account receivables management

Input provided by

Frank Blair, Ed Erway, Rhonda Killingsworth, Craig Rogers, Carrie Rudzik, Pam Ryan, Diane Ward

IT Strategy

1. "Always On" Computing
2. Data as a strategic asset
3. Electronic health record
4. Integration and interoperability of electronic systems
5. Support growth and outreach
6. Unified communications
7. Usability of installed systems
8. World-class IT service delivery Elaine Younce

Supply Chain Strategy

1. Warehouse automation
2. Pick list automation

3. PYXIS
4. Decision support system
5. Standardization
   Input provided by: Lorra Miracle

EHR & BIG DATA: - BASIC ARCHITECTURE [HEALTHCARE SUPPLY CHAIN AND REVENUE CYCLE]

[Examples From: HEALTHCARE SUPPLY CHAIN CONSOTIUM: Department of Supply Chain Management W.P. Carey School of Business Arizona State University]

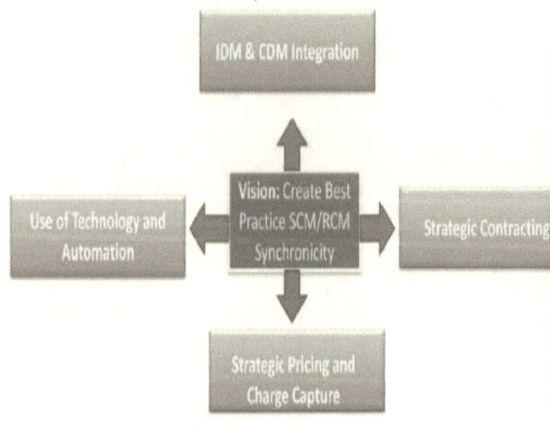

IDM & CDM Integration

SOURCE: Healthcare Supply Chain Consortium
    Figure 16

Successful management of supply chain and revenue cycle requires appropriately and accurately connecting key people and processes. Crucial to this management is a clean IDM. To optimize reimbursements and revenue, reimbursable supplies of the IDM must be linked to procedures in the CDM.

By establishing links between supplies and procedures, the process of tracking supplies, as important assets, is facilitated from acquisition to reimbursement. Thus, supply chain information technologies and decision support systems can be leveraged to help hospitals establish and ensure the linkage of the supply chain and revenue cycle.

Margins can be improved via SCM/RCM integration with a concentration on four important categories: (i) IDM/CDM Integration (ii) Strategic Contracting (iii) Strategic Pricing and Charge Capture, and (iv) Use of Technology and Automation. The optimization of operating margins calls for consideration of the cost of patient care and practices and processes utilized to bill for that care. Successful implementation requires accurate charge capture, inclusive billing, and uniform exchange of information with the IDM and the CDM.11 11 John Napiewocki and Anne Uruburu. "Margin for Improvement." *Healthcare Financial Management.* Feb 2005, 59, 2. Pg. 46

IDM & CDM Integration

Integration of IDM and CDM requires several essential components and strategic selection of key supplies and procedures in the linkage process:

Clean data files with current data and consistent item names and codes are necessary. Chargeable supplies that are not listed in the IDM should be identified and efforts should be taken to ensure supplies used in procedures are represented in CDM. The use of an updated, clean IDM can be helpful in updating and maintaining a current CDM. Ensuring accurate pricing reflective of costs Ensure charge codes for chargeable supplies are consistent with IDM coding. A template listing all supplies used in each targeted procedure is a helpful tool in the integration process. During the IDM/CDM integration process, it is also beneficial for hospitals to define appropriate new parameters for profit and loss reporting. Through integration of the IDM and CDM, hospitals can better account for chargeable supplies, which will increase supply accountability, reimbursement and decrease revenue leakage.

The IDM and CDM are reviewed on a daily basis at CHW to ensure that chargeable items are added to the corporate standard CDM and linked in Lawson. Additionally, CHW has incorporated its CDM with the item add process so that any time there is a new product introduced, adding it into the CDM is a mandatory step. The item is then coded as either chargeable or non-chargeable so that they can be easily identified. Reflecting the importance of managing the revenue cycle, there is also one corporate FTE, within the corporate CDM team, at CHW that is dedicated to the review and maintenance of the standard supply CDM. This FTE also does spot audits of facility charging practices.

At this time, JCL feels that they have a minimal level of SCM/RCM integration. JCL has a number of initiatives aimed towards improving the SCM/RCM integration as they estimate it costs $53 to re-work a claim, with some claims not even worth that amount. Abrazo has linked its patient accounting and billing systems to facilitate direct communication. Abrazo does this to leverage their IT systems to better capture otherwise potentially lost revenue. All three systems acknowledge the need for a clean, standardized, and linked IDM/CDM, but it is a significant challenge to accomplish. Decision-making at the hospital level rather than the system level perpetuates the problem of integrating the factors associated with margin management.

Abrazo Health Care [CASE STUDY] - Study Findings

Integration

The Vice President of Supply Chain at Abrazo Health is responsible for six hospitals and twenty physician clinics in Arizona. He reports to the CFO at Abrazo Health. Recently, the VP of Supply Chain has created a strategic plan for supply chain that aligns corporate (Vanguard Health Systems) and regional strategies to services lines. Abrazo is in an early stage of integration of its supply chain with RCM. The system is currently working on a total of 41 initiatives to integrate the Supply Chain Management and Revenue Cycle Management, of which 38 are scheduled to be implemented during 2012. Many of these initiatives focus on commodity management, physician preference item (PPI) standardization and purchased services and re-processing efforts. The integration process is being led by the VP of Supply Chain in collaboration with the head of finance.

Standardization

Vanguard Health Systems has a common IDM shared across all five regions consisting of over 6,000 supply items. A number of Information Technology (IT) systems are used for management of IDM, including McKesson Pathways Material Management (PMM) for its Enterprise Resource Program (ERP) and MMIS, ECRI for contract utilization management, Hyperion for decision support and financial performance analytics. Abrazo also uses a number of available website tools from its GPO (HealthTrust Purchasing Group.) Inventory management within Abrazo is fragmented.

Rather than a regional warehouse, each hospital has its own central storeroom that is managed with min/max reorder points and department level storerooms that are parred three times per week. Abrazo has successfully transitioned to a strategic focus utilizing value analysis teams (VATs), as well as scrutinizing DRG and profitability data to standardize its PPIs and lower inventory costs. Also being evaluated is the feasibility of moving to a central distribution center for the entire region with Abrazo running operations themselves or through an outsourced model.

Information technology (IT) Solutions

Abrazo views its patient accounting and charging system, Siemens MS4, and its billing system, Xactimed, as tools for integration of SCM and RCM to maximize revenue recovery. Abrazo outsources to Avega Health Systems for benchmarking data at both the physician and DRG level. This information is procured through co-management agreements and savings are shared between physicians. Abrazo continues with its integration work, with both progress and challenges. According to the VP Supply Chain, "The system has not yet matured to a regional mindset. We are slowly transitioning contracting and decision-making from an individual facility level to a regional level."

John C. Lincoln (JCL) Health Systems - [CASE STUDY] - Study Findings

Integration

At JCL, supply chain leadership does not exist at the corporate suite (C-suite) level. The Director of Network Supply Chain reports to the Senior VP and CFO. The Director also works closely with the VP of Revenue Cycle Operations to ensure accurate charging through its IDM, which is standardized throughout the network and contains over 15,400 active items. JCL has a written strategic plan for supply chain management. The main objective of the plan is to "increase employee and physician awareness and accountability for optimal management of supply costs."

Standardization

Current plans include "optimizing the buying power of the Network through the creation of a structure that supports efforts focused on better product utilization, standardization, and the management of new products and technology. " Also "decreas(ing) product expenditures by selection of the most effective and economical quality product based on trial and evaluation methods."

Information Technology (IT) Solutions

JCL uses a number of IT solutions to manage its operations, including PeopleSoft for MMIS and ERP systems and GPO provided analytical tools though Premier including MySpend, which offers benchmarking data, and Clinical Advisor. JCL is currently working on an initiative to transition from its current HIS system to Epic. Management at JCL believes that this change will bridge current gaps in performance. JCL uses PeopleSoft and At Par for inventory system management, a perpetual inventory model that is broken down by each business unit. JCL undergoes a physical count and adjusts its inventory levels annually. JCL uses VATs in an attempt to support standardization for its supplies. Additionally, a number of physician champions have been recruited to help with clinical resource utilization for selected Diagnosis Related Groups (DRG). There are no physician incentives or formalized gain-sharing approaches to support standardization at this time.

PART IV

[EHR: ACA - MEANINGFUL USE AND RELATED SHORT TERM FINANCIAL BENEFITS TO HEALTHCARE ORGANIZATIONS]

"To improve the quality of our health care while lowering its cost, we will make the immediate investments necessary to ensure that within five years, all of America's medical records are computerized ... It just won't save billions of dollars and thousands of jobs – it will save lives by reducing the deadly but preventable medical errors that pervade our health care system."

By: Honorable President Barack H. Obama [2009]

USA- INVESTMENT
[EHR]

Health Information Technology for Economic and Clinical Health (HITECH) Act of the American Recovery and Reinvestment Act (ARRA) (Blumenthal, 2011)
- Incentives for electronic health record (EHR) adoption by physicians and hospitals (up to $27B)
- Direct grants administered by federal agencies ($2B, including $118M for workforce development)

[CNN.COM]

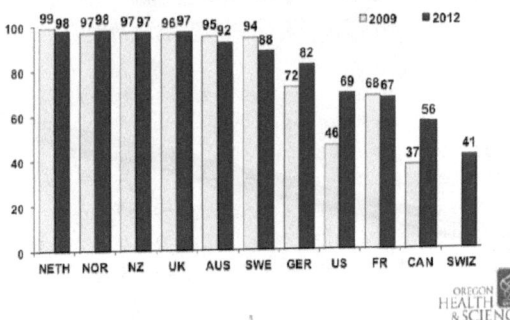

Figure 17

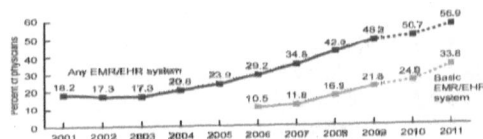

Figure 18

Although advanced functionality is less common (Schoen, 2012)

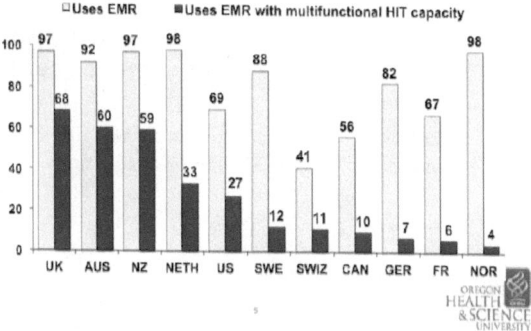

Figure 19

But the US healthcare system is still in need of fixing

- Recent IOM report (Smith, 2012) analyzes data to find annual
  - $750B in waste (out of $2.5T system)
  - 75,000 premature deaths
- Sources of waste
  - Unnecessary services provided
  - Services inefficiently delivered
  - Prices too high relative to costs
  - Excess administrative costs
  - Missed opportunities for prevention
  - Fraud

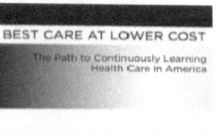
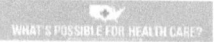
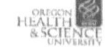

Figure 20

Health information technology (HIT) is part of solution

- Systematic reviews (Chaudhry, 2006; Goldzweig, 2009; Buntin, 2011) have identified benefits in a variety of areas
  - Although 18-25% of studies come from a small number of 'health IT leader" institutions

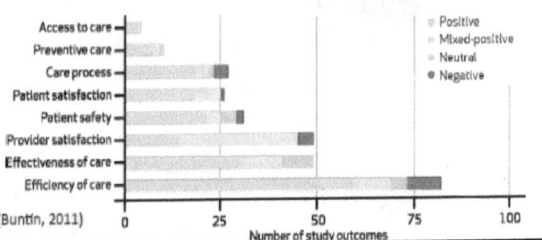

[Source: Oregon Health Science University]

Figure 21

IOM schematic for the learning healthcare system (Smith, 2012)

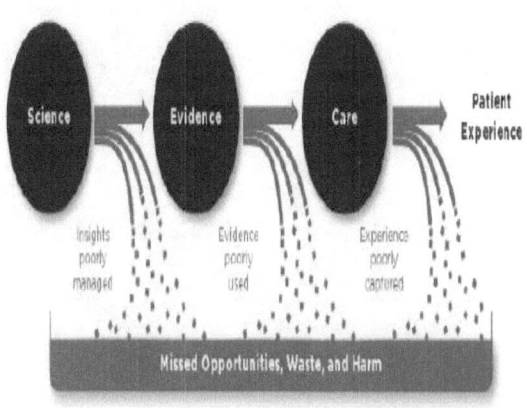

[Source: Oregon Health Science University]

Figure 22

Levels of BI (Adams, 2011)

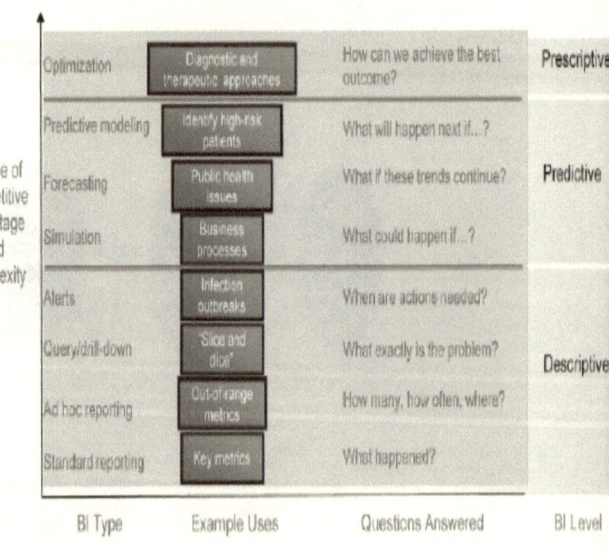

[Source: Oregon Health Science University]

Figure 23

PART IV

"HITECH Act § 13101 (amending the Public Health Service Act) (HITECH Act added 3000(5), which is now codified in scattered sections of 42 U.S.C.):

Health information technology is defined as —hardware, software, integrated technologies or related licenses, intellectual property, upgrades, or packaged solutions sold as services that are designed for or support the use by health care entities or patients for the electronic creation, maintenance, access, or exchange of health information.‖ 42 U.S.C. § 300jj(5); *see* AM. MED. ASS'N, Health Information Technology, http://www.ama-assn.org/ama/pub/physician-resources/health-information-technology.page (last visited May 12, 2011) (defining health information technology); CONG. BUDGET OFFICE, *supra* note 8, at 1 (stating EMRs are the primary health IT packages to send and receive data electronically).

HITECH Act §13101 (amending the Public Health Service Act) (HITECH Act added section 3000(13), which is now codified in scattered sections of 42 U.S.C. section 201):

A —qualified electronic health record‖ is: An electronic record of health-related information on an individual that – (A) includes patient demographic and clinical health information, such as medical history and problem lists; and (B) has the capacity – (i) to provide clinical decision support; (ii) to support physician order entry; (iii) to capture and query information relevant to health care quality; and (iv) to exchange electronic health information with, and integrate such information from other sources.

Evolution of Electronic Medical Records: From Pulp to Digital:

EMRs are longitudinal electronic records that contain patient health information, such as demographics, medications, allergies, medical history, immunizations, vital signs, and notes regarding past clinical encounters. EMRs fall under the broader category of Health Information Technology (—HIT), which also includes hardware and software used to collect patient data. EMRs contain information that a doctor or hospital staff member enter, and they are generally distinguishable from personal health records (—PHRs), which contain information that primarily the patient enters and documents. Not only do EMRs contain statistical data and information, but they also serve as a means of communication among health care providers, as a basis for planning future patient care, and as a means of protecting the legal interests of patients. Physicians and hospitals generally favor the implementation of EMR systems because they help streamline workflow, make patient information more readily accessible, reduce delays in communication, reduce errors, save money, and improve overall patient management.

    EMRs have come to the forefront of health care over the past several decades, as the United States has increased its desire to create a more efficient, cost-effective, secure, and accurate health care system. The rows and rows of paper medical records lining shelf upon shelf in doctors 'offices are all too familiar: the manila colored folders with the bright colored labels on the edge with last names and patient numbers. Such paper-based records are a physical manifestation of all of a patient's medical information. Information distilled in paper has limited abilities because only one person can have access to that record at any given time; labor costs are higher because greater resources are needed to copy, fax, store, and retrieve these records; and paper charts are difficult to scan to identify patient characteristics or statistics quickly and methodically. The push for greater implementation of EMRs has recently gained increased attention in the media due to President Obama's Administration's vigorous promotion of health care reform, particularly the Administration's emphasis on implementing EMRs to improve health care services and reduces costs.

A computerized record to contain health data, however, is hardly a new concept. The concept of computerized medical records developed in the late 1960s and early 1970s when both Lockheed Corporation and IBM suggested that computer records would increase quality of care and reduce paperwork. Yet, physicians remained hesitant to adopt this unproven, slow, expensive, and unreliable technology because the financial benefits were not evident. But, by the 1980s, EMR technology markedly evolved, as computer networking became widespread and data interchange standards became necessary for health care. Furthermore, federal governmental policies and research indicating EMRs could reduce the cost of health care also shaped the increased promotion and steady improvement of EMR technology during the 1980s.

Unfortunately, although technology was improving and EMRs were gaining widespread attention, the pressure in the health care industry to reduce costs dampened motivation to invest in expensive systems. In the 1990s and early 2000s, Presidents Bill Clinton and George W. Bush both touted the move from paper-based medical records to their electronic counterparts to provide a health system that allowed for greater efficiency, cost savings, decreased errors, and increased portability.

President Bush asserted the move from paper-based to electronic medical records would reduce medical costs by roughly twenty percent and would —help change medicine and save money and save lives. Most recently, the Obama Administration has been very vocal about the implementation of electronic medical records and the beneficial impact such records will have on national health care. The enactment of the American Recovery and Reinvestment Act of 2009 (—ARRA‖), the Health Information Technology for Economic and Clinical Health Act (—HITECH Act), and the Patient Protection and Affordable Care Act of 2010 (—PPACA), demonstrate the Obama Administration's strong commitment to improving health care and its particular focus on the implementation and use of electronic medical records.

A. Efficiency and Portability

Paper-based records hinder the effortless transferability of information from one physician's office to the next because they are bulky, must be physically present, and do not facilitate the smooth transition and physicians 'access to information. Further, using paper-based records may subject patients to increased risk of preventable errors when presenting themselves to various physicians and care facilities. This increased risk stems from the fact that the numerous doctors and care facilities do not have completely integrated information about the patient's prior medical encounters. On the other hand, EMRs increase efficiency because information is readily transmitted and accessed throughout the world via interconnected networks. A nationally connected health information network would also allow physicians to treat patients quickly without needing to restart the collection of a patient's entire medical history over and over again, regardless of where a patient moves or travels.

Greater accessibility to medical records results in greater efficiency because a doctor can quickly retrieve a patient's comprehensive medical history in seconds, without sifting through years of paperwork in a medical file, thereby enabling the doctor to make more informed and timely decisions. Moreover, increased coordination of information between health departments and organizations may additionally serve as a way to detect emerging health epidemics and to preserve medical records in the event of natural disasters.

B. Reduced Medical Errors

Electronic medical records are praised for reducing medical errors. Medical errors pose not only significant costs but also serious health risks, including death. In fact, medical error is estimated as the eighth leading cause of death in the United States, resulting in roughly eight million outpatient incidents and one hundred thousand deaths each year. Many medical errors are manual errors caused by humans working with paper-based records, including mishandled patient requests, inaccurate medical information, mislabeled specimens, misfiled or missing charts, improper dosages, duplicative testing, lack of information being entered, and more. As such, switching to electronic medical records and e-prescriptions can remedy such errors. Estimates suggest EMR adoption has the potential to save over four hundred thousand lives through improved disease prevention and management. Transcription error risks decrease and the expediency of transmitting medical and prescription orders increases when the orders and medical records are computerized. Errors may also be reduced by superior and more thorough information contained in EMRs and through the information technology (—IT) prompts that assist physicians in diagnosing patients.

C. Cost Savings

The health care sector could save between 81 and 162 billion dollars through national adoption and appropriate use of EMRs. Currently, administrative costs associated with health care often comprise between twenty-five to thirty percent of all health care costs.

Therefore, many of the administrative costs, which are based on the time it takes for administrative staff to transcribe physician notations, file records, process orders, and file claims, could be limited, thus greatly reducing the time spent on administrative activities and resulting in significant health care savings.

The Healthcare Information and Management Systems Society Electronic Health Record Association (—HIMSS), compiled statistics on the improvements and operational efficiencies health care provider organizations experience using electronic health records. The hospitals, physicians, and clinics that participated in HIMSS' research, which notably have all adopted EMRs, demonstrated quality improvements derived from implementing the EMRs, while also increasing output and patient satisfaction.

Moreover, operational efficiencies, the majority of which are administrative in nature, result in significant cost savings. Savings include reduced transcription costs, lessened malpractice insurance expenses, increased savings from decreased labor and supply costs for chart maintenance, diminished payments for medical records storage space, lowered turnaround time in prescription and medical orders, freed up funding through condensed administrative staff, eliminated radiology film costs, and improved accounts receivable turnaround times. Additional benefits and future cost savings may result from implementation of EMRs, but significant amounts of money must first be spent to implement these HIT systems, and many physicians 'offices cannot afford to implement the necessary infrastructure.

Risks Associated with Electronic Medical Records

A. Privacy and Security Concerns

EMRs provide many apparent benefits stemming from ease of transferability and portability, but these benefits are not without adverse consequences: EMRs also create significant privacy, confidentiality, and security risks. Privacy and security are primary patient concerns because health information technology has the ability to make medical information far more accessible and more easily transferable.59 Medical records contain sensitive information about patients, including details concerning interactions patients have with physicians. Consequently, proper security of such information is integral to ensure patient confidentiality; however, the federal privacy statutes that have been promulgated on this issue have not been as effective as intended. In 1996, Congress enacted the Health Insurance Portability and Accountability Juliana Bell, Comment, *Privacy At Risk: Patients Use New Web Products to Store and Share Personal Health Records*, U. BALT. L. REV. 485, 489 (2009) (maintaining disclosure of medical information can lead to embarrassment, job loss, health care fraud, ostracism, and difficulty obtaining health insurance if not properly secured); Colin P. McCarthy, Note, *Paging Dr. Google: Personal Health Records and Patient Privacy*, 51 WM. & MARY L. REV. 2243, 2248-49 (2010) (noting medical records contain a wealth of personal, financial, medical, and social data, as well as administrative information like consent and authorization forms); Steward, *supra* note 13, at 493 (discussing the critical information stored in medical records, and the need to adequately protect the information and address privacy concerns because ―[c]confidentiality is essential to effective health care‖); *see also* Gotkin v. Miller, 379 F. Supp. 859, 863 (E.D.N.Y. 1974) (describing information stored in medical records). The court stated: [A] medical record in the hospital or the physician's office is far more than a series of entries reporting diagnoses, doctor's orders and actions taken pursuant to such orders. In the hospital setting the record is a complex of communications between health professionals, including a written history and physical progress notes, nurses' notes, consultations, lab reports, operation summary, discharge summary and the like.

During the course of a particular hospitalization the record may include a wide spectrum of speculation and observation as the various members of the health team contribute thoughts and observations that lead eventually to the final diagnosis. If not properly explained, many of these entries could be exceedingly disturbing to a patient already apprehensive. *Gotkin*, 379 F. Supp. at 863. Act (—HIPAA) to address privacy concerns related to health information. Under HIPAA, certain covered entities were to implement safeguards to —protect the confidentiality or integrity of medical information stored in electronic records and integrated information systems against reasonably anticipated threats.

While HIPAA was a first step toward safeguarding patient information, and brought the issue of medical privacy to the forefront, it was not highly effective.64 By 2008, five years after the government began officially enforcing HIPAA, approximately 34,000 complaints of privacy violations were lodged. Today, medical identity theft is on the rise because the increasingly high cost of health care creates an incentive for people to steal identities to obtain health insurance. As more people are unable to afford to pay for health care, the amount of fraud and medical identity theft will continue to increase. Estimates claim three to ten percent of national health care spending is lost to fraud and abuse, equaling between $75 and $250 billion lost each year; accordingly, without adequate privacy protections in place, EMRs could exacerbate this problem.

Though HIPAA did not set forth specific guidelines for privacy and was not particularly effective, it brought privacy concerns to light and led to other legislation; in addition, it prompted the federal government assigned the Department of Health and Human Services (—HHS) with the duty of creating privacy rules. The Health Information Technology for Economic and Clinical Health Act (—HITECH Act), which was adopted to promote the meaningful use of health information technology and enacted under the American Recovery and Reinvestment Act (—ARRA), has imposed the most significant privacy and security regulations for the health care industry and its related business partners since HIPAA was adopted.

Specifically, the HITECH Act extends the complete privacy and security provisions of HIPAA to business associates of covered entities, thus eliminating one of HIPAA's limitations, and the HITECH Act introduces a structured approach to handling privacy and security breaches, increases civil and criminal penalties for breaches, imposes new notification requirements on covered entities, and applies to paper, electronic, and oral forms of information. The HITECH Act also provides consumers the right to obtain an electronic copy of their protected health information from HIPAA covered entities that use or maintain EMRs.

The recently enacted Patient Protection and Affordable Care Act of 2010 (—PPACA) further builds upon the provisions of the HITECH Act and HIPAA, emphasizing the importance of ensuring privacy and security of electronic medical records; specifically, the Secretary of HHS is required to ensure that all data collected are protected under privacy protections at least as broad as those protections promulgated under HIPPAA and the HITECH Act. As such, in September of 2010, Secretary Kathleen Sebelius, the Secretary HHS, adopted recommendations to effectuate PPACA's mandate. The recommendations significantly improve privacy and security of data and encourage greater state efforts to promote privacy and security of data. *[Source: Journal of Health & Biomedical Law [2011]]*

B. Pay-for-Performance

Pay-for-performance (P4P) programs are common financial incentive paradigms that emerged more definitively in 2000, in recognition of increasing health care costs and consumer demands for higher quality care. The concept of P4P is based on the idea that giving providers monetary rewards for providing quality care will improve the overall quality of medical care. By more closely aligning compensation with quality improvements, P4P programs reward doctors that keep their patients healthy, instead of providing rewards based on the number of patients seen and treated.188 P4P incentives are alternatives to fee-for-service programs that generally encourage ineffective and poor quality service because no mechanism exists to reward future health benefits. Insurance companies, government purchasers such as Medicare and

Medicaid, private employers, and health plans all sponsor P4P incentives.

In a similar vein as P4P, some policy makers have explored additional methods to incentivize physicians to adopt EMRs including looking to hospitals to financially support physicians. HHS issued exceptions to the federal physician self-referral and anti-kickback laws, opening the door for hospitals to assist in subsidizing physicians for the upfront and ongoing costs associated with EMR technology and support services; however, few hospitals have actually provided such subsidization for physicians. Not only would hospital subsidies provide incentives for physicians, but the subsidies would additionally lead to greater interoperability of systems because hospitals would be promoting the EMR systems they utilize and ensuring that physicians could integrate seamlessly with that system.

The underlying goal of reducing the financial burden for physicians through hospital subsidization, however, could actually increase the burden for many physicians. A physician closely aligned with the EMR system of one hospital may face increased costs by adapting records of patients treated at other unaffiliated hospitals with differing systems, or if the physician changes hospitals, the physician may also confront additional costs.

While initially a beacon of possibility, the P4P program is rapidly becoming the dodo bird of the health care industry. With the federal government allocating millions of dollars to assist with EMR implementation, as well as providing incentives through ARRA and other legislation, the majority of insurance companies no longer see the value in offering the P4P incentives. Accordingly, only a few contracts with payors will still have these P4P provisions written into them. Due to the difficult task of securing funds from federal government subsidy programs, physicians need greater financial incentives to adopt EMRs, such as higher reimbursement rates, or other subsidies to offset initial capital investments."

[Journal of Health & Biomedical Law [2011]]

PART V

[EHR: ACA – Meaningful Use and Sustainable Long Term Benefit To the Healthcare Industry]

"The Office of the National Coordinator for Health Information Technology (ONC) and the Centers for Medicare & Medicaid Services (CMS) offer multiple resources on their websites to help health care providers become meaningful users of certified electronic health record (EHR) technology. Below is a list of the resources available on meaningful use, Medicare and Medicaid EHR Incentive Programs, and the EHR certification process.

Meaningful Use and Medicare and Medicaid EHR Incentive Programs:

Meaningful Use Overview: http://www.cms.gov/EHRIncentivePrograms/01_Overview.asp

Path to Payment: http://www.cms.gov/EHRIncentivePrograms/10_PathtoPayment.asp

PowerPoint Presentation on Medicare and Medicaid EHR Incentive Programs Final Rule: http://www.cms.gov/EHRIncentivePrograms/Downloads/EHR_Incentive_Program_Agency_Training_v8-20.pdf

Timeline for Medicare and Medicaid EHR Incentive Programs: http://www.cms.gov/EHRIncentivePrograms/Downloads/EHRIncentProgtimeline508.pdf

Being a Meaningful User of Electronic Health Records: http://healthit.hhs.gov/meaningfuluse/provider

Meaningful Use Specification Sheets: http://www.cms.gov/EHRIncentivePrograms/Downloads/EP-MU-TOC-Core-and-MenuSet-Objectives.pdf

Flow Chart to Determine Eligibility for Medicare and Medicaid EHR Incentive Programs: http://www.cms.gov/EHRIncentivePrograms/downloads/eligibility_flow_chart.pdf

Webinar for Eligible Professionals on the Medicare and Medicaid EHR Incentive Programs: http://www.cms.gov/EHRIncentivePrograms/55_EducationalMaterials.asp

Certification Programs

Certification Programs Overview: http://healthit.hhs.gov/certification

Standards and Certification Criteria Final Rule Fact Sheet: http://healthit.hhs.gov/standardsandcertification/factsheet

HITECH Temporary Certification Program for EHR Technology Fact Sheet: http://healthit.hhs.gov/tempcert/factsheet

Temporary Certification Program Final Rule Frequently Asked Questions: http://healthit.hhs.gov/tempcert/faqs

Permanent Certification Program: http://healthit.hhs.gov/permcert/factsheet

Certified Health IT Product List: http://healthit.hhs.gov/chpl

Privacy and Security

Building Trust in Health Information Exchange: http://healthit.hhs.gov/buildingtrust

Health Information Privacy and Information on HIPAA: http://www.hhs.gov/ocr/privacy

Additional Resources:

ONC has also funded 62 Regional Extension Centers, located across the country, to offer customized, on-the-ground assistance for providers who need help adopting and meaningfully using certified EHR technology. For more information, visit http://healthit.hhs.gov/rec."

[Source: The Office of The National Coordinator for Health Information Technology.]

Electronic Health Records Incentive Payments for Eligible Professionals

"The Medicaid Electronic Health Record (EHR) Incentive Program provides incentive payments for Medicaid eligible professionals (EPs) who adopt, implement, upgrade, or meaningfully use certified EHR technology in their first year of participation in the program, and successfully demonstrate meaningful use in subsequent years.

For the Medicaid EHR Incentive Program, an EP must be one of the following five types of Medicaid professionals: physicians, dentists, certified nurse-midwives, nurse practitioners, and physician assistants practicing in a Federally Qualified Health Center (FQHC) or a

Rural Health Center (RHC) led by a physician assistant.

Note: Hospital-based EPs are generally not eligible to participate in the EHR Incentive Programs. The only exception is that Medicaid EPs practicing predominately in an FQHC or RHC are not subject to the hospital-based exclusion.

EPs may not receive EHR incentive payments from both the Medicare and Medicaid programs in the same year. In the event an EP qualifies for EHR incentive payments from both the Medicare and Medicaid programs, the EP must elect to receive payments from only one program and may only switch after receiving an incentive between the two programs once, and not after 2015. Furthermore, an EP who selects Medicaid must only receive incentive payments from one state in any payment year.

The Medicare Electronic Health Record (EHR) Incentive Program provides for incentive payments to Medicare eligible professionals (EPs) who are meaningful users of certified EHR technology. Under the Medicare EHR Incentive Program, an eligible professional is defined as one of the following five types of professionals:

1. Doctor of medicine or osteopathy
2. Doctor of oral surgery or dental medicine
3. Doctor of podiatric medicine
4. Doctor of optometry
5. Chiropractor

These professionals are eligible for incentive payments for the "meaningful use" of certified EHR technology, if all program requirements are met. Hospital-based EPs are not eligible to participate in the Medicare EHR Incentive Program. An EP is considered to be hospital-based if the EP furnishes 90 percent of his or her services in a hospital inpatient or emergency room setting. EPs may not receive

EHR incentive payments from both the Medicare and Medicaid EHR Incentive Programs in the same year. In the event an EP qualifies for EHR incentive payments from both the Medicare and Medicaid programs, the EP must elect to receive payments from only one program.

After an EP qualifies for an EHR incentive payment under one program but before 2015, an EP may switch between the Medicare and Medicaid programs one time. Upon switching programs, the EP will be placed in the payment year the EP would have been in had the EP not switched programs. For example, if an EP decides to switch after attesting to meaningful use of certified EHR technology for a Medicare EHR incentive payment for the second payment year, then the EP would be in the third payment year for purposes of the Medicaid incentive payments.

The 2014 Edition S&CC final rule completes the Office of the National Coordinator for Health IT's (ONC) second full rulemaking cycle to adopt standards, implementation specifications, and certification criteria for EHR technology. This final rule complements the newly released Centers for Medicare & Medicaid Services (CMS) final rule which establishes Stage 2 of the Medicare and Medicaid Electronic Health Record (EHR) Incentive Programs, updates Stage 1, and includes other program modifications.

The 2014 Edition S&CC final rule reflects ONC's commitment to reduce regulatory burden; promote patient safety and patient engagement; enhance EHR technology's interoperability, electronic health information exchange capacity, public health reporting, and security; enable clinical quality measure data capture, calculation, and electronic submission to CMS or

States; and introduce greater transparency and efficiency to the certification process."

[Source: The Office of The National Coordinator for Health Information Technology.]

PART VI

[EHR: - And the Future of Health Care: Discussions and Conclusion]

The insights gained from data through BI - Advanced Analytics using current and historical data [BIG DATA & DATA WAREHOUSES etc.] hold a myriad of great promises that has even proven themselves in many industries. These have given them lots of potential leverages that has not only helped some failing ones survived but significantly improved their bottom lines as well. Many industries from marketing to Banking & Insurance and Education has seen many advantages with enough evidence to justify their prominence and a business tool that has come to stay. For how long though will depend on time and their essence, for which we will leave for posterity to judge.

In my opinion, integrating such gems in business and operational systems anywhere [Any Industry] will help reduce the apparent and hidden risks in decision making and resource allocation etc, in managing the quality of related outcomes. A lot of other business conveniences can also sky rocket with such marriage of BI & Analytics using such requisite data from related infrastructures and systems. The competitive edges such advertences can potentially produce could only lead any business to great success and the lack of it to, extinction even. In other words, it is always a must have even for their survival, not to talk even further than that.

The sunk cost of the needed infrastructure and systems can be huge upfront, but affordability has nothing to do with its relevant and urgent need. Though the cost is high, depending on the business needs and size, it can also be mitigated by integrating with existing systems with an affordable pathway to the ends any entity seeks. Like Rome was not built in a day, a comprehensive plan is all that is needed, with enough time to implement depending on available resources and resource projections. This though should be done with an eye on the Industry and competitive elements within them, making sure one does not lag far behind to be left in the dark.

There is also a need to give room for a learning curve, and enough resources and patience for the learning and adaption process.

The inertia resulting from anxiety and resource crunch, as is apparent even in the Healthcare industry, cannot compare with the apparent and future benefits when the dust settles. It is therefore a must have, either than a should or want to have. Want and should have little to do with it. It is simply a do or die. You do not do, unless you are fed up with living, [A Joke].

As expressed earlier in the book, quality management is tied to how close expected outcome ties in with the observed. This can potentially get much closer with the right approach, such as the suggested framework [ASSPSC] within which BI & Analytics fits very well as well as Six Sigma and other already known related industry tools, used in managing business actions from decisions to outcomes, with an eye on expected quality standards. That should also be done well, with the knack for detail and meticulous business processes.

The eye though, should be on the outcome, not the processes alone. The processes however should be adapted with enough flexibility to steer it in the direction of the outcome, using existing tool in SIX Sigma, Business Process reengineering and the myriad of tools out there. The advised flexibility however does not suggest any reckless adaptation pathways etc. It is only necessary because the best can even be enhanced if time and purpose calls for it, not change for itself sake.

As has been presented, BI and analytics is quite young in healthcare, yet has made enough strides more so than their older cousins. It still has a lot more to offer if well integrated and redesigned if necessity asks for, to brighten it's superior opportunity cost and make it even better.

With the state of the healthcare industry and its dismal outcome indexes, from cost, operational, customer satisfaction, clinical, morbidities and mortality etc., such technology adaptation holds a great, potential in improving not only the odds, but significantly improving the bottom lines of most entities in the Industry, as well as ultimately engendering the most fort after, wellbeing and happiness of patients via the enjoyment of the longevity of their good health, as opposed to the misery of the pain and suffering that comes with disease, and also the scarce resources allocated to such interventions needed to mitigate such risks, which could have been used for other life essentials like food, transportation, education and shelter, and also with the added confidence which most Obese patients lose, due to substandard societal perceptions of their physique which undermines their self esteem etc., and other adverse psycho-social nuances and more.

Positive outcomes necessary to avert such results in healthcare can only be achieved via the most needed collaborative engagements with industry partners, and sharing of related data and insights to come with the needed harmonized solutions, which best suites their multilateral interest. Through a very well thoughtful integrated approach and thinking process, compromising conveniences, value for value, to get the best practical outcomes, for which the interest of the patient should be paramount.

Such engagements and the needed requisite data could have never been possible without the Electronic Health Record Systems and related infrastructure, some of which are in place and others being built and implemented.

The inceptives given via ACA [Affordable Care Act] to accelerate the most needed pace is worth commending. And as such will thank legislators on both side of the isle, in the house of congress and senate [USA] who made it possible, and also for President Barack Obama, and subordinates at the executive branch of the US Government, for finally signing it into law to make it happen to bless many in the country.

[Deux Lux Scientiae]

References

- [1] Bhatnagar, A. (2009). Web analytics for business intelligence. Online, 33(6), 32-35
- [2] Baars, H., & Kemper, H. (2008). Management support with structured and unstructured data - an integrated business intelligence framework. Information Systems Management, 25(2), 132-148. Doi: 10.1080/10580530801941058.
- [3] Lamont, J. (2006). Business intelligence: The text analysis strategy. KM World, 15(10), 8-10.
- [4] Brannon, N. (2010). Business intelligence and E-discovery. Intellectual

Property & Technology Law Journal, 22(7), 1-5.

- [5]Chaudhuri, S., Dayal, U., & Narasayya, V. (2011). An overview of business intelligence technology. Communications of the ACM, 54(8), 88-98. doi:10.1145/1978542.1978562.
- [6]De Voe, L., & Neal, K. (2005). When business intelligence equals business value. Business Intelligence Journal, 10 (3). 57-63
- [7]Kudyba, S., & Rader, M. (2010). Conceptual factors to leverage business intelligence in healthcare (Electronic medical records, six sigma and workflow management). Proceedings Of The Northeast Business & Economics Association, 428-430.

- [8]Glaser, J., & Stone, J. (2008). Effective use of business intelligence. Healthcare Financial Management, 62(2), 68-72.
- [9]Sahay, B.S., & Ranjan, J. (2008). Real time business intelligence in supply chain analytics. Information Management & Computer Security, 16(1), 28-48. doi: 10.1108/09685220810862733.
- [10]Reinschmidt, J., & Françoise, A. (2000). Business intelligence certification guide. Retrieved August 10, 2011, from http://www.redbooks.ibm.com/pubs/pdfs/redbooks/sg245747.pdf.

- [11]Fickenscher, K.M. (2005). The new frontier of data mining. Health Management Technology, 26(10), 26-30.
- [12]Giniat, E. (2011). Using business intelligence for competitive advantage. Healthcare Financial Management, 65(9), 142, 144, 146.
- [13]Hocevar, B., & Jaklic, J. (2010). Assessing benefits of business intelligence systems - a case study. Management: Journal of Contemporary Management Issues, 15(1), 87-119.
- [14]International Organization for Standardization (ISO/TC 215). (2005). Health informatics — electronic health record — definition, scope, and context. Geneva, Switzerland: ISO. Retrieved from

http://www.openehr.org/downloads/standards/iso/isotc215wg3_N202_ISO-TR_20514_Final_%5B2005-01-31%5D.pdf

- [15]Agrawal, R., Grandison, T., Johnson, C., & Kiernan, J. (2007). Enabling the 21st century health care information technology revolution. Communication of the ACM, 50(2), 34-42.
- [16]Bonney, W. (2012). Enabling factors for achieving greater success in Electronic Health Record initiatives. In E. Conchon, C. Correia, A. Fred, & H. Gamboa (Eds.), Proceedings of HEALTHINF 2012: International Conference on Health Informatics (pp. 5-11). Vilamoura, Algarve, Portugal: SciTePress.

- [17]Watkins, T.J., Haskell, R.E., Lundberg, C.B., Brokel, J.M., Wilson, M.L., & Hardiker, N. (2009). Terminology use in electronic health records: Basic principles. Urologic Nursing, 29(5), 321-327.
- [18]Halley, E., Sensmeier, J., & Brokel, J. (2009). Nurses exchanging information: Understanding electronic health record standards and interoperability. Urologic Nursing, 29(5), 305-314.
- [19]Coiera, E., Westbrook, J.I., & Wyatt, J.C. (2006). The safety and quality of decision support systems. Methods of Information in Medicine, 45(Suppl. 1), 20-25.
- [20]Wadsworth, T., Graves, B., Glass, S., Harrison, A., Donovan, C., & Proctor, A.

(2009). Using business intelligence to improve performance. Healthcare Financial Management, 63(10), 68-72.

- [21]Jung, E., Li, Q., Mangalampalli, A., Greim, J., Eskin, M.S., Housman, D., Isikoff, J., Abend, A.H., Middleton, B., & Einbinder, J.S. (2006). Report Central: quality reporting tool in an electronic health record. AMIA Annual Symposium Proceedings. 971.
- [22]Smith, G., Hippisley-Cox, J., Harcourt, S., Heaps, M., Painter, M., Porter, A., & Pringle, M. (2007). Developing a national primary care-based early warning system for health protection--a surveillance tool for the future? analysis of routinely collected

data. Journal of Public Health, 29(1), 75-82.

- [23]Safran, C., Bloomrosen, M., Hammond, W., Labkoff, S., Markel-Fox, S., Tang, P.C., & Detmer, D.E. (2007). Toward a national framework for the secondary use of health data: An American medical informatics association white paper. Journal of the American Medical Informatics Association, 14(1), 1-9.
- [24]Teasdale, S., Bates, D., Kmetik, K., Suzewits, J., & Bainbridge, M. (September 2007). Secondary uses of clinical data in primary care. Informatics in Primary Care, 15(3), 157-166.
- [25]Yeoh, W., & Koronios, A. (2010). Critical success factors for business

intelligence systems. The Journal of Computer Information Systems, 50(3), 23-32.

- [26]Jordan, J., & Ellen, C. (2009). Business need, data and business intelligence. Journal of Digital Asset Management, 5(1), 10-20.
- [27]Follen, M., Castaneda, R., Mikelson, M., Johnson, D., Wilson, A., & Higuchi, K. (2007). Implementing health information technology to improve the process of health care delivery: A case study. Disease Management, 10(4), 208-215.
- [28]Information Systems Analysis 488 Topic: Decision Support Systems Randall E. Louw 1074205 University of Missouri St. Louis Prof. Vicky Sauter

http://www.umsl.edu/~sauterv/analysis/488_f02_papers/dss.html

- [29]"BI-Big Data Analytics and Health Care – A Review
  Kwasi Yeboah-Afihne, Dinesh P Mital and Shankar Srinivasan
  Department of Health Informatics,
  Rutgers School of Biomedical Sciences – SHRP, 65
  Bergen Street, Newark, NJ-07067, USA
  E-mail: kwasi_afihene@yahoo.com, mitaldp@umdnj.edu, srinivsh@umdnj.edu

  I J C I H I : Vol. 6, No. 2, July-December 2013, pp. 41-49 Care – A Review 41
  © Serials Publications, ISSN: 0973-7413

- [30]"Importance of health information technology, electronic health records, and continuously aggregating
  data to comparative effectiveness

research and learning
health care. Miriovsky BJ. Shulman LN. Abernethy AP. Journal of Clinical Oncology. 30(34): 4243-8, 2012 Dec 1. UI: 23071233".

- [31]"Cost-outcomes focus is essential for ACO success.
Greenspun H. Bercik W. Healthcare Financial Management. 67(2): 96-102, 2013 Feb. UI: 23413676".
- [32]"Big data in health care. Schouten P. Healthcare Financial Management. 67(2): 40-2, 2013 Feb. UI: 23413667.
- [33]"Maximize performance with BI and big data.
Comparative analytics enables organizations to benchmark performance against their peers. Sanderson M. Health Management Technology. 34(1): 18, 2013 Jan.

UI: 23420987.
- [34]"Emerging directions in analytics. Predictive analytics will play an indispensable role in healthcare transformation and reform. Edelstein P. Health Management Technology. 34(1): 16-7, 2013 Jan. UI: 23420986.
- [35]"Accountable care and data analytics emerging in healthcare. White SE. Taylor LB. Journal of Ahima. 83(11): 56-8, 2012 Nov-Dec. UI: 23210300.
- [36]"Making advanced analytics work for you. Barton D. Court D. Harvard Business Review. 90(10): 78-83, 128, 2012 Oct. UI: 23074867".
- [37]"Big data: the management revolution. McAfee A. Brynjolfsson E. Harvard Business Review. 90(10): 60-6,

68, 128, 2012 Oct. UI: 23074865".
- [38]"Great timing for a smart company. As analytics becomes all-important, a highly capable data analytics firm is well-positioned for the future. Hagland M., Healthcare Informatics. 29(6): 34-5, 2012 Jun-Jul. UI: 22896940".
- [39]"Research and analytics in combat trauma care: converting data and experience to practical guidelines. Perkins JG. Brosch LR. Beekley AC. Warfield KL. Wade CE. Holcomb JB. Surgical Clinics of North America. 92(4): 1041-54, x, 2012 Aug., N.I.H., Extramural. Research Support, U.S. Gov't, P.H.S. UI: 22850161"
- [40] "Importance of health information technology, electronic health records, and continuously aggregating data to comparative effectiveness research and learning health care. Miriovsky BJ.

Shulman LN. Abernethy AP. Journal of *Clinical Oncology.* **30**(34): 4243-8, 2012 Dec 1. UI: 23071233".

- [41] "Cost-outcomes focus is essential for ACO success. Greenspun H. Bercik W. *Healthcare Financial Management.* **67**(2): 96-102, 2013 Feb. UI: 23413676".
[3] "Big data in health care. Schouten P. *Healthcare Financial Management.* **67**(2): 40-2, 2013 Feb. UI: 23413667.
- [42] "Maximize performance with BI and big data. Comparative analytics enables organizations to benchmark performance against their peers. Sanderson M. *Health Management Technology.* **34**(1): 18, 2013 Jan. UI: 23420987.
- [43] "Emerging directions in analytics. Predictive analytics will play an indispensable role in healthcare transformation and reform. Edelstein P.

Health Management Technology. **34**(1): 16-7, 2013 Jan. UI:23420986.

- [44] "Accountable care and data analytics emerging in healthcare. White SE. Taylor LB. *Journal of Ahima.* **83**(11): 56-8, 2012 Nov-Dec. UI: 23210300.
- [45] "Making advanced analytics work for you. Barton D. Court D. *Harvard Business Review.* **90**(10): 78-83, 128, 2012 Oct. UI: 23074867".
- [46] "Big data: the management revolution. McAfee Brynjolfsson E. *Harvard Business Review.* **90**(10): 60-6, 68, 128, 2012 Oct. UI: 23074865".
- [47] "Great timing for a smart company. As analytics becomes all-important, a highly capable data analytics firm is well-positioned for the future. Hagland M.,*Healthcare Informatics.* **29**(6): 34-5, 2012 Jun-Jul. UI: 22896940".

- [48] "Research and analytics in combat trauma care: converting data and experience to practical guidelines. Perkins JG. Brosch LR. Beekley AC. Warfield KL. Wade CE. Holcomb JB. Surgical Clinics of North America. **92**(4): 1041-54, x, 2012 Aug. , N.I.H., Extramural. Research Support, U.S. Gov't, P.H.S. UI: 22850161".
- [49] ONC Fact Sheet: 2014 Edition, Standards & Certification Criteria (S&CC) FINAL RULE: The Office of the National Coordinator for Health Information Tech.
- [50] CMS: EHR Medical Electronic Health Record Incentive Payments For Eligible Professionals : Last Updated: May 2013
- [51]Medicaid Electronic Health Record Incentive Payment for Eligible Professional Last Updated: May 2013.

- [52]eHealth University Centers for Medicare & Medicaid Services: An Introduction to: Medical EHR: Incentive Programe Eligibility Professionals: CMS
- [53] eHealth University Centers for Medicare & Medicaid Services: An Introduction to: Medical EHR: Incentive Programe Eligibility Professionals: CMS
- [54] Unofficial Recitation of Portions of 42 CFR Part 495 and 45 CFR PART 170 #

www.ingramcontent.com/pod-product-compliance
Lightning Source LLC
Chambersburg PA
CBHW020857180526
45163CB00007B/2542